Run *LIKE A* MOTHER

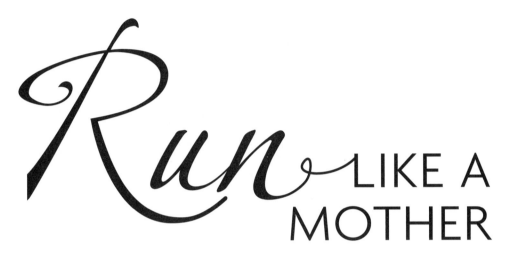

Run LIKE A MOTHER

How to Get Moving—
and Not Lose Your Family, Job, or Sanity

by Dimity McDowell and Sarah Bowen Shea

Andrews McMeel
Publishing, LLC
Kansas City · Sydney · London

Andrews McMeel Publishing, LLC
an Andrews McMeel Universal company
1130 Walnut Street, Kansas City, Missouri 64106

www.andrewsmcmeel.com

ISBN: 978-0-7407-8535-1

Library of Congress Control Number: 2009940823

10 11 12 13 14 SHD 10 9 8 7 6 5 4 3

ATTENTION: SCHOOLS AND BUSINESSES
Andrews McMeel books are available at quantity discounts with bulk purchase for educational, business, or sales promotional use. For information, please e-mail the Andrews McMeel Publishing Special Sales Department: specialsales@amuniversal.com

CONTENTS

INTRODUCTION

October 10, 2005

To: Sarah

From: Dimity

So on my walk this morning, I'm thinking: marathon in spring 2007? Wanna? It was drizzling, like it did in NYC in 1997 (!) and made me nostalgic for running 26.2 while my feet are sopped.

To: Dimity

From: Sarah

So are you talking you and ME doing marathon, or just you!?

To: S

From: D

I'm thinking we run it together. Well, maybe not exactly together, as you'll be way faster than me, but we will keep each other accountable for training (more for my benefit than yours), then meet up in a cool city and run, run, run. No pressure: There's over a year to commit. :)

Just heard the peanut's heartbeat—what a sweet sound. Yay.

To: D

From: S

YAYYYYYYY! Heartbeat!!!! Soooo excited for you!

I'd LOVE to do a marathon "with" you—although you will be the speedier one. I tell you, I am SLOW now. While I was carrying the twins, my pre-pregnancy running partner dusted me. She's 48 and just did her first marathon (Portland) . . . 3:56. She qualified for Boston. It's KILLING me!

Oh, marathon MUST be flat or flat-tish and in a city west of Chicago, if not even closer.

October 31, 2005

To: S

From: D

OK, you have some qualifications, but I think we can work around them. Let's place it on the back burner, and revisit next fall.

And, BTW, I gotta say, the Nike Women's Marathon sounds really appealing. I know it's in the fall, and I doubt I would be ready next fall, but maybe fall 2007? I'm thinking if I run sub-4:30, I'll be feeling like Tegla Loroupe. The other good thing about Nike: It's also got a half-marathon. Not that I won't aim for the 26.2 stars, but just in case.

April 10, 2006

To: S

From: D (5 days away from due date with second kid)

Just took Dharma for a walk. 45 minutes is my max now, and it's mostly on flat roads. Can't WAIT to get back into shape. Still thinking about Nike marathon in '07. Wish it could be this year, but I'm kidding myself.

To: D

From: S

Babe, I am not ready for marathon this fall! Fitness is coming back, but slowly. I'm in ma-thetic shape (ha ha!). I hear you on being READY to not be preggo anymore!

May 30, 2006

To: S

From: D

Went for my first run. Pathetic. Five minutes of "running" (at a 10 mph pace, being optimistic) and 5 minutes of walking x 4. It really hurt. Decided to wait until post—July 4th to try again, and try to do more fast walking/hiking in the meantime. Thought about pitching Nike Women's Marathon to *Runner's World* though: Do you think they'd bite?

August 23, 2006

To: S

From: D

Had EXCELLENT run last night—overcast, in the low 70s, hadn't done cardio in about 4 days (so I had energy), listened to Dixie Chicks and Lucinda Williams. Ran for 50 minutes, with a 1-minute break about minute 26 (to switch from the Chix to Luci). Marathon seemed possible.

Also got my brain thinking about angle we could use:

Long-distance training partners. How slow was your ma-thetic pace again? Thinking if we're about the same pace, we get put on the same training plan/same workouts, and we can bitch about them and tell how we squeeze workouts in, etc. Could also see how two people on the same plan produce different results. Thinking we type you as competitive, me as laid-back. (I'd rather win silver than gold. Honestly.)

December 8, 2006

To: S

From: D

I've been running more: 4 x 45 minutes this week, and am feeling good. Let's get a marathon pitch to *RW* by end of first week in January? Sorry I haven't moved on it.

To: D

From: S

Yes, let's pitch *RW*. My only "concerns" now are that Nike Women's Marathon and Head of the Charles are the same weekend! But let's HOPE we have such problems: having to decide b/t the two. Please, I haven't done anything either! But I FULLY intend to any day now, I swear.

New rule: no apologies.

A few phone calls follow, during which Sarah and Dimity don't think a plain old marathon is compelling enough to pitch to *Runner's World*, but the Transrockies, during which teams of two cover 125 miles in 6 days, is being held for the first time that fall, and we pitch it. They bite, and we freak out: No way can we train for 125 miles.

To: Tish, Executive Editor at *Runner's World*

From: Sarah

Dimity and I are psyched *RW* is so excited by our Transrockies proposal . . . but, as you might guess, we let our enthusiasm get the better of us when we put it together. After sending it off without much thought about how long 125 miles really is, and how much we'd have to train to get there, reality set in. Separately, we both realized the training for the race—and the race itself—would do us (and our marriages!) in. Images of disgusting houses, disgruntled husbands, and kids eating cheese pizzas for dinner every night because we're too tired to make anything else were enough to make us reconsider.

But we don't want to abandon the idea totally—just downsize it a bit. We were thinking we could run the Nike Women's Marathon in October. Because 26.2 isn't, well, 125—and the train-wreck appeal isn't there—we could factor our mentalities into the equation and either play them up as they naturally are or train to balance them via a sports psychologist or similar expert. (Something like, Dimity has to actually go at a pace that hurts, while I have to try to chat up at least one person a mile.)

Anyway, we look forward to hearing from you—heckling included.

To: D

From: S

Twinge of regret/sadness went thru me when I just hit "send" on our reply to Tish. But, honestly, at this point in our lives, the race would have done us in. Otherwise, our next joint assignment would be, "Physical studs, mental wrecks: dealing with divorce and kids while being in the best shape of our lives."

February 9, 2007

To: D/S

From: Tish

Hi you two,

Why am I not surprised?

Maybe because I went for a run yesterday with a fellow editor who was talking up the race. I said, "Oh, I want to do that." Then he said, "You can! I can get you an entry no problem!"

Wait, hold on. Twenty miles a day, at altitude, a week away from home, not to mention the training, childcare, and full-time job? Um. Never mind.

> D/S send a few e-mails, pitching and pleading for a Nike Women's Marathon. Tish says she already has a writer on the case.

February 22, 2007

To: D/S

From: Tish

Did I say no?

I meant yes. We had a meeting this morning, and talked it through, and you're on for the Nike Women's Marathon in October. (Now don't go saying you can't do it.)

How's that sound? You still up for this?

Lemme know.

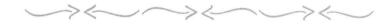

And that, in an extended e-mail nutshell, is how this book began. We both got across the finish line in 2007, and as we trained and raced and wrote about our experience, we realized that there's a revolution going on around the country. It might not be on par with, say, Tiananmen Square circa 1989, but marathon moms—amazing, multitasking women who work, parent, wife, and, in their spare time, also run, whether it's around the block or along a 26.2-mile marathon course—are popping up everywhere. Evidence? In between the 2 hours and 23 minutes it took Paula Radcliffe, mother to then 9-month-old Isla, to win the 2007 New York City Marathon and the 5 hours, 29 minutes it took Katie Holmes, aka Mrs. Tom Cruise and mother to Suri, to cross the line, countless (unphotographed but not uncelebrated) marathon moms also went the distance.

But we're not just running in New York City. We're running around Denver's Washington Park; we're navigating the Wildwood Trail in Portland, Oregon; we're training with three of our new best friends in Austin for the Rock 'n' Roll Marathon; we're pushing double-joggers in Cleveland as we funnel Cheerios to our children to keep them happy during a 30-minute run; we're heading out with a neighbor in Springfield and wondering whether we can make it to the end of the cul-de-sac and back. We're running to beat cancer or to raise money for a sister-in-law fighting it. We're running to process a bad day and, in doing so, make it better. We're running to set a good example for our children. We're running to feel lean, strong, empowered, and graceful. Although we're not running the country (yet), we're definitely getting in shape to do so.

As our assignment morphed from a magazine assignment to a book contract, we immersed ourselves in the ad hoc community of mothers who run. We reached out to hundreds of running mothers and got their feedback on everything from what hurt most on their first post-birth runs to how they justify taking time away from their families for a 12-miler. The responses, sprinkled throughout the book, solidified what we already knew: Mothers who run are opinionated, funny, and smart women. In other words, mothers who run are women we are always psyched to spend some time with.

Run Like a Mother is a conversation between us. But not just the two of us. All of us, from Paula to Katie and beyond: fast, slow, motivated, not so much, marathoners, sprinters, trail runners, and stroller pushers. Our chat takes place over the following 26 chapters, with a .2—a nod to the final stretch of the marathon—in between each chapter for a break of sorts.

We hope that you enjoy reading the discussion as much as we liked creating it. When you are through, let's make running mothers a more formal community. Find us at runlikeamother.com, at our Run Like a Mother: The Book group on Facebook, or at runmother @gmail.com. Let's keep this dialogue going . . . and going, and going.

—Dimity and Sarah

01

RUNNING FOR OUR LIVES: **PART I**

By Dimity

Around 5:30 this morning, a minor war is brewing. The combatants? Dimity v. Dimity. In one corner, standing solo and alert, is the athlete in me, the one who thrives on the routine and afterglow of a good sweat. "Get up," she commands. "Get your butt up, out of bed, and on a run. You know you won't regret it." She isn't lying. An early morning run lubes and recalibrates both my mind and my body. After a run, the day ahead—which, like most, begins around 6:30, packing a lunch for my picky daughter, and includes two work deadlines, a grocery store excursion, and swimming lessons and ends around 10 P.M., emptying the dishwasher—feels effortlessly conquerable. In fact, after 5 miles at 5:30 A.M., any day is a downhill coast. Still, it's hard to motivate when it's dark outside. So last night, in order to mitigate any seemingly valid excuses to stay warm and cozy, I piled my running clothes in the downstairs bathroom to be able to slip out without waking my family. Well, most of my family. "Kick me out of bed when my alarm goes off," I instructed my husband, Grant, before closing my eyes.

In the other corner, drooling profusely on the pillow, lay the rest of me: a freelance writer who jams 40 hours of work into 20; a mother of Amelia, a 6-year-old who, like most, asks more questions than a *Jeopardy* contestant, and Ben, a 3-year-old whose idea of fun is ramming cars into his sister's head; a wife who wants enough energy at the end of the day to have a conversation with her husband beyond, "Did you feed the dogs?" (Oh yeah, I've got two dogs, too.) "Hit snooze, stupid," says my more reasonable half. "You can run later today, or tomorrow, or never. Aren't you busy and stressed enough as it is?" With NPR droning in the background, the two parts of me bicker like my kids over the last lime popsicle. (Grant, who, like most husbands, happily honors every request I make of him, is no help this morning. He didn't even stir when the alarm blared.)

Only half-conscious, I still am well aware of who is going to win this war. I hit snooze. Once. Then I fall out of bed and down the stairs and grab a banana on the way to the bathroom. I slip off my PJs, pull my sports bra over my head, and fumble with my balance as I jam my feet through the lining of my running shorts. I stuff my iPod earbuds in my ears and the banana in my mouth, and I groggily head out into the cool spring morning.

The first steps always feel painfully rusty, no matter what time of day it is. These ones are no different. I fantasize about climbing back under the covers with my workout clothes on. I think about cutting my run short by at least 2 miles. I wish running didn't mean so much to me. I wonder why I can't live like the rest of the world, who thinks a 7 A.M. alarm is really aggressive. But then Gwen Stefani starts proclaiming that she ain't no Hollaback Girl, and I start to feel her groove. A mile passes, then two, and the sun starts poking up from behind the mountains. On a slight downhill, my pace easily picks up. "I'm alive!" I gush along to a rocker-chic cover of the Neil Diamond song, fully aware of how corny I'm being and fully not caring.

But it's the truth: For an overstressed, overtired, overextended mother, there are few other sensations that rival a delicious run. Once the sweat starts running down my temples, I daydream, analyze, smile, wonder, channel something cosmic. I feel alive and, perhaps most importantly, like myself again.

The funny thing is, I'm not really a runner. Standing at almost 6 feet 4 inches, I've never once been mistaken for one. My first memory of the sport is the Presidential Physical Fitness Test we were subjected to in middle school. I could pound out sit-ups as capably as anybody, and I willingly shook uncontrollably as my chin barely cleared the pull-up bar, but the running tests? Ugh. I would've pulled out the popular excuse most of my friends did—I have my period—to get out of the dreaded mile, except that I hadn't gotten my first one yet. So I laced up my Tretorns and loped around that dusty, gray track four excruciating times. I was out there so long, I was sure I had missed my bus ride home. I think I beat only one other kid: Bill, a pudgy boy with gapped teeth who, as usual, was wearing penny loafers because he never remembered to bring his tennis shoes.

The 100-yard dash was up the next day. Despite the significantly shorter distance, that event was even more painful because Mr. Blanski, the gym teacher, singled me out, which, for a teenage girl, is a fate worse than getting your first period at school while you're wearing white pants. For the 100, we raced in pairs. Within seconds of Mr. Blanski blowing his whistle, Brooke, a super-coordinated gymnast, was steps in front of me. "C'mon, Dimity," Mr. Blanski bellowed. "Can't you use those long legs for something?" My cheeks turned red from embarrassment, not effort, but I managed to maintain enough composure so that I didn't trip over myself, a regular occurrence in those days.

I realized then that my long legs were not made for running.

I stumbled onto the college rowing team—as it turns out, long legs are an asset in crew—and we ran for cross-training during the winter. Let me rephrase: I jogged/walked/jogged/walked for a couple months before I got to the point where I could "run" (read: a 12-minute mile) the hilly 3-mile loop around campus. Although my aerobic system was able to handle the load of running much better than it used to be, I hardly embraced the sport. I always felt sluggish. I was absolutely positive the effort I had to muster up to propel myself forward was much, much harder than what any of my twenty teammates had to create. They made it look so much easier than how it felt to me.

Long after graduation, though, I was still tromping on the pavement. Simplicity and efficiency, two of running's hallmarks, are hard to trump when a) you're broke and living on bagels in New York City as an editorial assistant; b) you get a raise, enough to buy a road bike, but are frightened to ride it very far lest you get a flat tire; c) you pop out two kids and, for the next 5 years or so, have exactly 30 minutes to exercise daily; or d) all of the above. I pick "d."

Fifteen years later, I've run infinitely more steps than I ever took strokes in rowing. Even though I've survived two marathons, six or eight or ten half-marathons—as you'll discover, I'm not a number person—and even more shorter races, I'll be honest: On some days, I still despise running. And why not? It's hard. It hurts my knees. It kills my ego: I'm the passee way more often than passer. It makes my butt and thighs jiggle. It robs my breath and makes my heart work ridiculously hard. It feels so belittling that all those thousands of miles I've run up to this point can sometimes seem to amount to absolutely nothing.

And yet, on days when I'm sure somebody has traded the insoles in my shoes for 5-pound weights, I'm still happy to be there for one simple reason: I am alone with my thoughts and tunes. These days, when I can't go to the bathroom without an audience, I appreciate the solo aspect of running more than any other item on its long list of benefits. When I run, I'm not a mother or a wife or a writer. There's no whiny child pleading, "Momma, can I just watch TV? Pleeease?" after she's already been plugged into the tube for an hour. No insensitive editor telling me, "Dimity, this is good, but you'll need a new angle, ten more studies, and five more expert quotes. Does tomorrow sound doable?" There's no husband who can inexplicably tune out all canine and child chaos out as soon as he checks his e-mail or opens the newspaper.

When I run there's just me, with no agenda, putting one foot in front of the other, relishing the simplicity and grace of the motion. The trip-trap, trip-trap of my heels lull me into a dreamy space where the reality of my ulcer-inducing life doesn't faze me. Running is more powerful than any drug I've taken, and I'm fairly certain it's the elixir that has allowed me to maintain a sliver of my former self—and my sanity.

This morning, I pass three other runners, women who seem like me. We're no longer in the prime of our single years, when a self-induced hangover—not a sick kid or a BlackBerry back-and-forth with a boss at 11 P.M.—quashed a morning run. We've left behind our easy-to-be-fit years, when getting ready to sport a swimsuit simply meant cutting down on the Coors and picking a pattern from J. Crew, not doing a cayenne-pepper cleanse and spending hours in a dressing room trying to find a sassy tankini that doesn't scream "I'm a mother with the stretch marks to prove it." As I run by the other women, I gasp out a quick "Morning." The brevity of my greeting belies the admiration I have for my fellow runners, both this morning and universally. I respect—and relate to—you because you're out here, like me, at a ridiculously early hour, getting it done.

There are millions of you out there in our tribe, and as hokey as it sounds, I know, if we randomly struck up a conversation, we'd soon discover we're both runners and think, "I could be her friend." Running connects people like that. Whether you're huffing through 12-minute miles or ready to slash a 3:20 personal record (PR) in the Philadelphia Marathon, I sense a bond between female runners that is immediately present and surprising in its depth and intimacy. (My proof? Within minutes of running with a new friend, Amy, with whom I'd only e-mailed, we were talking husbands, jobs, and frustration like we'd known each other for years.) The link between mothers who run is even more overpowering: When you're commanding a ship of people who rely on you to sometimes obnoxious degrees, finding the time, energy, and inspiration to jump overboard and get out the front door alone can be as challenging as the run itself. Embracing—or at least grudgingly accepting—that challenge links us in meaningful, lifelong ways.

Surprisingly, for me, who went from a very reluctant runner to an often-still-have-to-convince-myself runner, the sport has become a way in which I define myself. Not in an "I'm a 3:15 marathon runner" way (as if!), but in the more substantial, intangible ways running permeates your soul. I don't doubt myself in tough situations because I am a runner. I feel almost invincible because I'm a runner. I have amazing friends—the kind I can call at 2 A.M. because I'm not sure if a 103-degree temperature warrants an ER visit—because I'm a runner. I have the guts to set seemingly impossible goals and then methodically work toward them because I'm a runner. I realize my limitations because I am a runner. I appreciate the strengths and accept the weaknesses of my body because I'm a runner. (OK, I'm still stubborn on the weakness part, as too many injuries illustrate.) I know how to keep on keeping on, even when I'm sure I've got nothing left to give, because I'm a runner.

Don't worry: I never think that profoundly as I wrestle my submissive half out of bed at the crack of dawn. All I really ask myself is, "Should I run today?"

The answer is always yes.

RUNNING FOR OUR LIVES: **PART II**
By Sarah

You know how it goes: You mention you've run a few marathons, and folks think you are some stud-runner. But when I also let it slip that I'm a mother of three young kids, including preschool twins, they look at me like I'm a supernatural being.

I'm never sure why that is. Do the child-free think caring for a child deprives you of the ability to put one foot in front of the other in a rhythmic fashion? Or that once you have a kid, you should resign yourself to a life of Lincoln Logs and Legos, forgoing any personal hobbies or interests you had in your pre-mommy life? Does mothering really drain all the energy out of a woman, leaving none for fitness, weight management, or competitive endeavors?

Nope. I have never seen motherhood and running as mutually exclusive.

In fact, I've become more athletic since having kids. I'm not sure why, but I think it might be like why I got better grades during rowing season in college (like Dimity, I rowed in college). The busier I was, the more focused I became. If I had only 2 hours after practice to translate a Mayakovsky poem from Russian to English and read three chapters of *Jane Eyre*, I'd hammer out my homework and then head to bed. If I had twice the time, I'd fritter the evening away at the library, talking to my boyfriend, and not be asleep until at least 1 A.M.

It's the same with my weekend life before I started a family: With no responsibility other than to wake up and eventually get to the grocery store, it was easy to let a Sunday slip by without exercising. (Ah, I fondly remember those days, when the alarm clock gathered dust on the weekends. Brunch didn't start until 11 A.M., which often led to window shopping and a pedicure, and then maybe a nap.) Now I know that if I'm not out the door by 8 A.M. on a Sunday, I'll never get in my 10-miler. There's no time to contemplate the logistics of a run. When you're a mom, it's now or never—even when "now" is often well before a day has had a chance to pink up.

There are a few other reasons why I am a more avid runner now that I'm a mom. There's the obvious: alone time. As dearly as I love my husband, Jack, and my three kids—big-sis Phoebe, 8, and 4-year-old twins John and Daphne—I would go berserk (bananas, nutty, insane, cuckoo, loco, pick your adjective) if I didn't get out of the house by myself almost daily. My (running) hat is off to moms who have the patience to spend every moment from sunup to sundown with their kiddies, but I am most definitely not one of those women. I need to get out and just be me, not the time-out-giver, snack-bestower, or boo-boo kisser. I want to be merely a woman in a running skirt, sweating out the stress so I can return ready for another trip to the playground.

Then there's pride. Being an athlete is a badge of honor I wear along with my H&M jeans and Anthropologie sweater. As much as I can't imagine life without Phoebe, John, and Daphne, I strive to have a separate identity from them. I guess I could cultivate myself as a gardener or flutist, but running just suits me. Now that my kids are finally beyond the cry–breastfeed–nap stage, even they realize I'm an athlete. It delights me when, as I tuck her in, Phoebe asks me how far I'm running the next morning. I chuckle when John refuses to hug me when I return after a run because, "Momma, you all wet."

Another side of pride? Being able to brag about my workouts and my race results. (Dimity, who can't remember whether her first marathon time was 4:32 or 4:23, insisted I get it out of the way in the intro, so here are my personal bests: 6:37 for the mile, 22:19 for 5K, 47:37 for 10K, 1:49 for the half-marathon, and 3:52 for the marathon.) Unlike the mom we carpool to school with, Molly, I don't wear my half-marathon medal and tee to Easter brunch (she'd just run the race the day before), but I love that she does. However, I do often manage to work a conversation around to running and casual mentions of my times. And God love Facebook: It gives me a whole new outlet for boasting. I'll 'fess up: There have been times at the track when I've needed some motivation to fire up my legs on a mile-repeat, and I've envisioned my status update on Facebook being, "Sarah Bowen Shea is a Boston qualifier." Anything to get the job done, right?

I also run to feel alive. To remind myself I am a corporeal being, that I have a body. To feel a chilly breeze on my bare legs, to feel sweat streaking down my brow, to feel my arms pump back and forth, to feel the soles of my feet hit the pavement, to feel my lungs suck in air. As a writer, I find it too easy to live life in my head, to feel like a brain with extensions (read: hands) tapping on a keyboard. And as a mother, I sometimes just feel like a mouth, saying "no" or "don't cry, you're OK" or "do you want a cheese stick?" When I run by myself, which is the majority of the time, I turn off my brain and my mouth. I used to tell myself I'd debate a problem or think up story ideas while running, but I've come to realize that never works. When I switch on my body to run, my brain shuts off. It flatlines. All my worries, internal debates, and concerns get tamped down by the rhythmic pounding of my feet. I love it.

When a fellow mother asks if I'm a runner, I'm more than happy to tell her, sometimes at length, I am. And when the conversation comes around to the trio of kids and a full-time job, she asks the inevitable, "How do you ever do it?" I launch into the logistics of running in the morning and planning races around school vacations, and she gets that stunned look in her eyes, like I'm accomplishing the impossible.

Far from it. I'm merely doing an activity that is as essential to my existence as food or water. There's no debate about whether to make time for running. I just do.

.2 SHOULD YOU RUN TODAY? **A QUIZ.**
By Dimity

Being wishy-washy about whether or not you should run simply wastes what little free time you have. To expedite your decision, take this quiz.

1 Your to-do list today:

   A Is bullet-pointed on a Post-it Note.

   B Fits on the back of a piece of your child's artwork.

   C Needs a paper clip to keep it from scattering everywhere.

2 Before bed last night you:

   A Took a bath, shaved your legs, exfoliated your body, mud-masked your face.

   B Brushed, flossed, and splashed clean water on your face: good enough.

   C Ripped off your shoes and pants, decided you didn't mind sleeping in a bra and collapsed under the sheets.

3 The last full meal you ate:

   A Contained at least three of the major food groups.

   B Was packaged in plastic and heated up in a microwave.

   C Was consumed over the steering wheel and, as such, dipping the French fries in ketchup was not an option.

4 Your sleep last night:

   A Started before David Letterman began and ended after the sun rose.

   B Included fewer than two get-ups for monster-under-the-bed checks, drinks of water, and the like.

   C Included at least one uninvited family member in your bed, and not enough personal space to find cool spots on the sheets when you needed them.

5 The last time you actually used your running shoes to accelerate was:

   A Easy: yesterday. Five miles, three of which were at tempo. You came home and logged it in your workout log.

   B Sometime between now and the day last week that had the same name as today.

   C To sprint after your child, who was tearing down the candy aisle, trying to escape with a 16-ounce bag of gummi bears.

6 Your mood today can be summed up as:

   A Sunshine, even on a cloudy day.

   B Fine. I'm pretty fine, really.

   C Don't talk to me; don't look at me; definitely don't ask me how I'm doing.

7 The last time you sat down in front of the television, you watched:

   A A marathon—*Project Runway*, *Law and Order*, *Desperate Housewives*, whatever— and you got through two episodes without interruption or falling asleep.

   B Larry King ask his guest three whole questions.

   C *Dora the Explorer*, as you tried to distract your daughter while clipping her nails.

8 The last time you listened to your own adult music was:

   A Another easy one: yesterday. Killers, Springsteen, Coldplay on a 5-mile run.

   B Does humming along with the Muzak version of Culture Club's "Karma Chameleon" in the supermarket count?

   C I'll tell you as soon as I get that annoying *Blue's Clues* theme out of my head.

9 Today, you're most looking forward to:

   A Tackling the PowerPoint presentation you've been putting off for days.

   B Assembling the ten-segment, multicolored caterpillar you saw in a parenting magazine and thought, "Finally. There's an arts and crafts project I could handle doing with my kid!"

   C Bed as soon as possible.

10 Truthfully, how much do you really want to run today?

   A Pick me! Pick me! Can I do some more mile repeats?

   B I'd be fine taking it, but I could also leave it.

   C My body barely has enough energy to smile and blink at the same time, let alone run.

Tally up your score and decide accordingly.

Mostly A's: Not necessary, but if you feel you must, head out. Just don't be too perky as you pass those having a harder time.

Mostly B's: You're not required to run, but you do have to sweat so your mood can either improve or plateau, not nosedive. And since running is the most efficient way to get the temples soaked, run.

Mostly C's: Don't go hard, and don't go long, but most definitely, *definitely go.*

02

MOTIVATION:
CREATING MY OWN STIMULUS PACKAGE

By Dimity

The life of a mother is a life of nonnegotiables. There's really no choice about cleaning up a puke-filled crib at 3 A.M. It's got to be done. Ditto for sending back field trip permission slips, feeding the class guinea pig your daughter volunteered to adopt for summer vacation, and ensuring your kid has some semblance of oral hygiene. At times, even sex seems mandatory, to remind your husband this half-crazed woman bobbing around the house is, in fact, his wife. Laundry can easily pile up, but at some point you have to suck it up and sort it; after all, even turning underwear inside out for a second wear has its limits.

So where does a run fit into a to-do list whose length makes the Constitution look like a Post-it Note? Or, more accurately, where do you find the energy and oomph to run? Unfortunately, the inspiration doesn't just magically appear one day like Oz's good witch Glinda: "Today, Dimity, you will instantly be bestowed with fresh legs and a willing mind," she says, waving her wand. "Run long and have a blast!" I wish.

Not to get all Richard Simmons on you, but in order to become a runner, you have to make a choice. And that choice is you: you over family, you over work, you over PTA and book club and being the parent volunteer on the field trip to the science museum. You have to decide you deserve to take enough time in a week—2 or so hours, at least—where running, and consequently you, is the priority. You have to believe that your mind and body are valuable enough to hire a babysitter so you can run or that a lunch hour is better spent on the treadmill than over the keyboard. You have to find ways to overcome inertia, minimize exhaustion, and overlook overscheduling so you can simply say, "Now it's time for me to enforce my own time-out." After you make that mental leap, you then have to realize that the initial complaints your body feels as you sputter into a rhythm are minor compared to the benefits you'll reap after your run.

Run LIKE THIS MOTHER
TO LOG OR NOT?

Every motivational guru offers up some variation of the same tip: Keep a workout log in which you write down when, where, how fast you ran, and how you felt. While I understand the rationale behind it—you can appreciate how much work you've done and tangibly see your improvement—I've never been able to embrace the log. It feels like another chore, and I'm just not that interested in reminiscing over a 6.3-mile run I did in drizzle with a sore hamstring on August 13, 2003.

But because I was writing a story about the 2007 marathon, I did keep a fairly consistent real log through my months of training (usually filled in weekly with data copied from my Garmin). I suffered a heel fracture early on, and spent much of my time on the bike, indoors, building up my cardiovascular base. On the plane headed to the race, I got a massive case of the doubts: Who trains for a marathon on the bike? I pulled out my log and studied each week and realized how much sweat I'd poured out in order to get to San Francisco. I wasn't totally at ease with the challenge ahead, but my log reassured me I'd done all I could.

But I haven't looked at it since.

Don't let a few creaks stop you. You have to trust that running will make you a more productive and pleasant person.

So instead of listing all the reasons why today is simply not the day for a run—it's too cold, life's not fair, your wand is missing—a better call is coming up with solid reasons why running is another nonnegotiable.

I'll start. Here are my top ten reasons for running, in order of importance:

1   The mental high I know I'll coast on after a workout, a wave powerful enough, most days, to combat my genetic tendency toward moderate depression.

2   The stream-of-consciousness river that appears about 10 (awfully slow) minutes into a run, then flows from one temple to the other. As my feet thud below me, in my head I carry out tough conversations I wish I had the guts to have for real; I imagine what my life would be like today if I were single and child-free (I'd be a much more prolific writer, I tell myself, and way more concerned with accessories); I relive childhood swim meets, a high school road trip to Kansas, and other random memories that make me smile; I fantasize about a house swap in

TAKE IT *From* A MOTHER
WHEN DO YOU PREFER TO RUN?

"6 a.m., from my front door: the kids are asleep, my husband is available if they need him, and I only have to shower once that day. Best way to start my day."

—ROBYN (runs "until my head is cleared of problems and I have plans of attack.")

"Morning. I enjoy my whole day so much more if I run in the morning. A good run clicks me into optimism mode."

—CHRISTINE (how long have you been a runner? 25 years. "OMG!")

"I wish I could run first thing in the morning so I could have it over for the day. But my body doesn't really produce 'productive' runs as far as speed or mileage—relative terms—until after lunch."

—PAMELA (runs on the road. "Treadmill? Sing me a lullaby now.")

"I run mostly on my lunch hour because I don't want to take time from my kids. My long runs are before noon on the weekends."

—MELANIE (favorite post-run treat: cheese, chocolate, and froufrou drinks.)

"If it's too hectic of a day to squeeze in a run, I'll get dinner prepared for my family, then head out after my husband gets home from work and they settle in to eat dinner."

—SUSAN (emergency TP during a trail race: flags marking the course. "When I confessed this to my husband, we laughed our heads off.")

"During the week, I run right after work at about 4:30. I know myself well enough that if I get in my car and drive home, I will not be running."

—WENDY (averages 75-80 miles a week.)

"I used to enjoy a nice run over lunch or after work. Now, as a mother, I find my days work best when I get all my me-time before the kids wake up. So I run at 5:30 A.M. or earlier. If you would've told me four years ago that's when I would be running, I would've told you you're nuts."

—KELLY (proudest moment: when her 3-year-old son came into the kitchen, pushing a doll in a stroller, and announced he was "going for a run.")

PRACTICAL *Motherly* ADVICE
TURN YOUR LIGHT FROM RED TO GREEN

I can dream up an excuse to skip a run as quickly as my kids fake-gag when I put broccoli on their plates. So I don't give myself the chance. I get up early, get it done, and don't have to spend the rest of the day fruitlessly searching for a valid reason (a hangnail?) to say, "Thanks, but no." In that early morning fog, my brain can't protest. It just goes along for the ride.

If you're not an early morning person, here are some other strategies that might give you the push you need:

♀ Don't give yourself an out. Bring your running clothes to work, change there, and drive to a park to run before you head home for the evening.

♀ Blare your favorite song before you change your clothes. You'll already be grooving before you get out the door.

♀ Get off the sidelines. If your kid has soccer practice, make sure his cleats are double-knotted, then take off for a run. When Amelia has a 45-minute swim lesson at the Y, I put Ben in the free childcare and head for the treadmill. Yes, I dread the 'mill, but I'll take it over watching 5-year-olds learn sidestroke.

♀ Become a prostitute—or at least pay yourself for your services. Not totally psyched to train for a marathon, I ponied up $1 for every mile I ran in preparation. I ended up with $742 and spent almost every penny on myself. Selfish? Yes. But also exactly what I—and my sad, stained wardrobe—needed. You don't have to be as indulgent as I was: Pay yourself a quarter for every mile; after ten runs, make a matinee date with a girlfriend; promise to make cupcakes with your kiddos after your 7-miler on Saturday.

♀ Find a running BFF. I can't overemphasize how helpful it is to have a sole sister, someone you know is counting on you to show up and make each step easier by chatting, laughing, or merely being by her side. Whether you're a stay-home mom or a worker bee, American motherhood can be woefully isolating; a standing social date, even if it does involve huffing and puffing, makes me feel like I'm part of the world again.

♀ Don't get runner's block. My most traveled route is one of convenience: It's exactly 4 miles, nearly flat, and out my back door. It works most of the time, but sometimes I don't want to know exactly how many steps (thirty-two, most days) are between the two bridge underpasses. When I get writer's block, I head to a coffee shop for a change of scenery. When I get runner's block, I go to a new trail, a set of masochistic hills, or a friend's tried-and-true route. Remembering whether I need to turn right or left at that corner makes the run go by so much faster.

♀ Create your own Hall of Fame. Angie, a mother of two, writes her finishing time and place on each race bib and pins them in her closet. Monica, another mom of two, puts them in her cubicle at work.

♀ Don't go. And then see how you feel. Chances are, you'll be out there tomorrow.

New Zealand; I figure out a tricky transition in a story. The best part about the mental float is I'm off the hook; my subconscious holds the remote control, so whatever gets served up, I enjoy.

3 Being able to drink a beer (or three), scarf a Twix at the movies, or order a bacon cheeseburger without (much of) a second thought.

4 The knowledge that my mileage translates to a body, a few joints excepted, that is a finely tuned, disease-fighting machine and will be around to kiss the delicious round parts of my great-grandchildren.

5 The soothing exhaustion a morning workout creates, which hits about 7 p.m., instantly slows me down, and has me in REM sleep by 9:30, max. When it appears, I forgo mundane duties— paying bills, picking up the house, sending ten more "urgent" e-mails—in favor of a rejuvenating bath, a long-overdue chat with my husband, or a brainless date with bad television.

6 The active lifestyle my kids think is the norm, not the exception, and will, fingers crossed, replicate in some form.

7 The mellow demeanor my post-run self brings to being a parent and spouse. I'm more patient, more engaged, and less quick to snap.

8   The very tangible, improving results that come with structured, consistent training. Nothing else in my life is as concrete and objective as those numbers.

9   Uninterrupted girlfriend time.

10   The sense of admiration I get when I tell people I've run two marathons. (They have no idea how doable it is.)

My number one reason to run—fighting off the blues—is what I'd call a tortoise: a sucker that will never die. Tortoise reasons, such as mental clarity and stress relief, provide plenty of impetus to get moving for a lifetime. There's never a day when I think, *Gee, I'd rather be more stressed* or *Wouldn't it be great to have my brain feel more braided?* I can also resort to hare reasons for inspiration, like the fact that last night I ate a piece of chocolate cake roughly the size of Ecuador, so today I've got 6 miles served up. Short-term prods, such as fitting into a bridesmaid's dress, are great for jumpstarting a program, especially for a beginner runner. You set a modest goal and, with a little dedication, get the results you wanted. Ultimately, though, the hares aren't sustainable because you're eventually able to slither into the taffeta, and then you're left with no immediate reason to run.

The good news, beyond the fact you looked kick-ass in the wedding pics, is that running has a sly way of getting under your skin. While you're all gung-ho, achieving the hare goal, you also stumble upon a few tortoises—an almost cosmic calm, a mind clearer than your skin has been in decades, jeans that aren't suctioned to every inch of your thighs—which are unexpected and more enticing than you ever anticipated. So enticing, in fact, you choose more often than not to keep going and going.

Truth be told, reminding myself of my tortoises doesn't jolt me out there; the irony of running is that when your body and spirit need it most, your mind wants to do it least. That said, no matter how bad my funk, I'll drag myself out there. I've proven to myself, again and again, I'll come out on the other side in a much better place.

After all, we know who eventually wins the race.

.2 THE DAY I BECAME A REAL RUNNER
By Sarah

I firmly believe I'm not a natural athlete. My husband, Jack, occasionally affirms that self-conceived notion when he tells me I'm the fittest one in our house, but he's the most athletically talented. (His cockeyed rationale has something to do with him playing baseball and football as a teenager, while I only played 2 years of high school tennis.) Now that I've admitted this, you shouldn't be surprised to learn I often look to others for validation. Don't get me wrong: I'm an outspoken woman with a bumper crop of self-confidence, but when it comes to defining myself as a jock, I look to others for an assessment.

By June 1998, I was training for my first marathon. At that point in my life, I'd been a fairly regular 4- to 6-mile runner for at least a decade. But the decision to tackle 26.2 miles all in one day made me feel like a poser, a wanna-be. Not like OshKosh, the genuine article.

After a 16-mile run one day, Jack and I headed to a backyard BBQ in a Chicago suburb. I didn't know many of the people, just a few of Jack's fraternity brothers. The father of one of Jack's buddies was there, the dad of a guy named Hanson Williams, who had been childhood friends with Tommy, another guest at the party. Turns out Mr. Williams was a man of few words until I arrived on the scene. He immediately walked up to me, looked me up and down—I was sporting khaki shorts because it was a muggy summer evening—and asked me, "What marathon are you training for?"

Me and marathon in the same sentence? And it was apparent I was a runner? I was floored: I'd never been sized up as a runner before. A swimmer or rower, yes, thanks to my broad back, and a hoops player because of my 5-foot, 11-inch frame, but never a runner. Mr. Williams and I proceeded to talk about running routes in Chicago and training plans for about 15 minutes. It turned out he was an avid runner who'd done plenty of marathons, including two Boston finishes. A lean, handsome man, he was an old-school runner who kept track of his lifetime mileage, which at that point was an awesome 44,000 miles.

Finally, all talked out of 26.2 details with the nontalker, I excused myself to grab a turkey burger and some potato salad. As I stood by the grill, Tommy rushed up to me, dying to find out what I'd talked about for so long with Hanson's dad. I told him we'd chatted about running. Tommy exclaimed he'd known Mr. Williams since he was a kid, yet the man had never spoken as many words to him in his life as he'd just said to me! I laughed along with Tommy, Hanson, and Jack about that one, but underneath I was so surprised and excited that a veteran marathon runner had spotted me as a kindred spirit. Maybe I wasn't a poser after all.

03

MENTAL TOUGHNESS: **TRAINING MY BRAIN**

By **Sarah**

A BIT OF A DISCLAIMER

Don't be tempted to skip this chapter, using the (lame) excuse that you're not fast or serious enough to worry about mental toughness. Like the scale of perceived physical exertion where a 1 means no prob and a 10 means big prob, there's a spectrum of mental toughness, and you and your running experiences fall somewhere in it. To my knowledge, no exercise physiologist has ever formalized it, so let's just say it goes from 0, "A pimple can sideline my running for a week," to 10, "If I don't puke, pass out, or both, I didn't give all I got." Dimity ranks about a 4. She pushes mildly during races but has never, and will never, vomit from physical effort, whereas I tend to be, um, more intense. I'd say about a 9. So don't think you have to be like me to consider yourself worthy of analyzing how your head affects your feet. Instead, know this: No matter where you fall on the spectrum, the stronger your head is, the better you'll be as a runner.

In almost every race I've ever run, my goal is to empty my proverbial tank. I tell myself to do so as I'm waiting on the start line, and I often chant it under my breath, mantra-like, during the race. Even Jack knows to yell it out to me from the curb—and has trained the kids to do so.

To me, there's always been something mythical about the idea of leaving everything out on the race course. Of crossing the line in an utterly depleted state. It makes me feel like an authentic athlete, like a real runner. I just had to know what it felt like.

Yet until the Eugene Marathon in Oregon in May 2009—25 years into my athletic career—my needle never touched "E." As hard as I tried to push myself to the brink, I inevitably pulled back, forever crossing the finish line with more in me. Sometimes I'd have only a few drops left, but it still wasn't empty. After a race, I always had to admit to myself I could have pressed down the accelerator harder than I had. Why didn't I push it to the floor? I was petrified I'd run out of fuel before reaching the finish line and be reduced to walking, which is the ultimate humiliation to me. A beyond-bonked finish would cast a klieg light on my greatest fear: being revealed as an athletic impostor, not a genuine player.

But not at Eugene. Nope, not at Eugene.

Eugene was my fifth marathon with the explicit goal of finishing in less than 4 hours. It had been my goal with the previous 4 attempts, but I believed this to be my final—and best—shot. As a 40-something mother of three, I knew my chances weren't as ripe as they'd been a decade before, when I ran my first 26.2. Also, this time I had the ultimate booster: Olympic medalist Lynn Jennings as a coach. Lynn and I had met through mutual friends and become good pals through several work projects. By the time I returned from my disappointing fourth marathon, she could see I had the passion to PR. I just needed to be honed. Not only did she generously give me customized workouts for free, but she also frequently did long runs or track sessions with me. And she got so deep inside my head, our joke became she had implanted a chip inside my brain.

Lynn had a canny sense of knowing how much I was capable of, then asking for just a bit more. I came to the more challenging workouts wearing a cloak of uncertainty over my technical tee and running skirt, yet up until April 8, I had consistently emerged triumphant. But on that Wednesday morning, less than a month away from M-Day, self-doubt echoed in my head as Lynn and I headed over to the track at the local high school. On tap: 6 miles of work, broken down as 1 × 1 mile, 2 × 2 miles, 1 × 1 mile. It was my first time doing 2-mile repeats; I didn't know what to expect. She set the bar high by admitting she wanted to do the 2-mile repeats in 15 minutes or less. I felt my stomach clench; 2 weeks earlier, we'd done 4 × 1 mile in times ranging from 7:30 up to 7:57. Lynn would never think poorly of me if I fell short of her high standards, but my pride hadn't let that happen—at least not yet.

Lynn and I alternated leads on laps, me taking the odd ones and her the evens. She took off on her first lap of the first 2-miler faster than usual, confirming my fear. Usually I didn't struggle to stay on her shoulder, but that morning I did. There were moments, especially on the curves, when I could feel her slipping away from me, and I had to mine a deep reserve to catch up with her on the straightaways. As I drove with my elbows and ordered my quads to fire harder, I also had to tamp down the self-doubt chatter in my head. Our time for that first 2-mile repeat was 14:54, with splits of 7:32 and 7:22.

As we continued around the track for an 800-meter recovery, with me gasping for full breaths, Lynn told me, "This is a workout elite marathoners do. Many runners would never be able to handle the task of 2-mile repeats. They don't have the mental skills to accomplish a workout like this. You do."

I let her comment sink in to my sweaty pores and worm its way into my psyche.

TAKE IT *From* A MOTHER
WHAT'S YOUR MANTRA?

"I am a strong, healthy mother of three."

—AMANDA (dream running date: "You stumped me. I really just like to run alone.")

"It's your head, not your body, that's hurting, so move it!"

—CHRISTINE (hopes to run another sub-4 marathon after her second kid is born.)

"The faster you run, the faster you're done."

—DANA (runs when her daughter is at ballet or kids are at tennis lessons.)

"Junko: You are an Ironman!"

—JUNKO (disclaimer: "I run marathons and have never finished an Ironman, but for whatever reason, it gets me going.")

"Kill the hill."

—KATHY (saying originated while running up four-block-long Haight Street Hill in San Francisco Marathon)

"What are you saving it for?"

—KELLI (ran her first half-marathon with her mother-in-law, only 6 months after she started running.)

"Don't think, just go."

—CYNTHIA (explanation: "I have found even the cleverest motivation speech composed the night before won't have a chance against the right brain's desire for more sleep at 4:30 a.m.")

"SHARP, which stands for Stay Here And Run, Princess."

—KRISTYN (explanation: "We have a SHARP television mounted in front of our treadmill, and one day, when I was having a hard time motivating, I thought about what those letters stood for.")

"I am a badass tri chick!"

—RAQUEL (avoids trails because "I trip over air.")

"Run with your heart."

—REBA (other motto: "Just keep running," adapted from Dori in *Finding Nemo*.)

"Suck it up."

—DIANA (doesn't run with her kids because "It would defeat the stress-reducing effect of a run.")

"Leave it on the pavement!"

—MELANIE (loves running by lakes, rivers, and oceans.)

"You are a warrior."

—KIM (started running at age 11. "I had to wear a scoliosis brace, and my doctor let me take it off for an extra hour daily if I was running.")

Soon after my breathing evened out, we kicked into our second 2-miler. I instinctively knew she wanted to beat the time of the first one. Sure enough, Lynn turned on the turbo-boosters as soon as she started leading the second of the eight laps. My mind scrambled, pinging me with thoughts of fear, doubt, and pain. Then, through the static, a line from the horror film *Poltergeist* zinged into my brain: "Walk toward the light, Carol Ann. Walk toward the light."

Let me explain. Jack and I bandy about that line when one of us has to make a difficult decision or feels inundated. The light, we assume, will show the way. Silly, I know, but it works for us—as it did for me that morning. Instead of giving in to the sense of being overwhelmed, I fired back and ran into the glow. We shaved 4 seconds off the clock, running 2 miles in 14:50. Not to be outdone, we then ran the final mile of the workout in 7:15. Elation fueled my shuffle home; I'd left all my physical energy on the track.

Come race day, under drizzly, gray clouds, I ran the first 3 or so miles at a smart, ease-into-it pace, then I put my foot on the gas. And left it there the rest of the way. In the week leading up to the marathon, I'd been scared and nervous about the pain and strain I'd feel, despite Lynn assuring me my body and mind were trained for the task. Now I believed her. I was comfortably running mile after mile at a pace between 8:32 and 8:47. My steps were fluid, not forced. Around mile 8, I yelled out, "I feel fantastic!" to our friends Amber and Angella, who were cheering me on.

The going got tough about mile 25, but I knew I had more in me to give. After all my hard work, I wasn't going to let myself once again taste regret over a few remaining drops at the finish line. Three months of Lynn's workouts had nudged me ever so slightly beyond my comfort zone, past what I thought I was capable of. They let me know I could keep pouring it on. So I did.

Then, steps before the 26-mile marker, my tank really, truly, finally, for the first time in my life hit empty. I felt such a dramatic shift in my energy level and my gait, I swear I heard an audible "click." The engine was officially dead. Ironically, it was almost exactly when my friend Ellison, nicknamed "E," ran past me and then turned back to urge me to keep up with her. I had the will to do so but no fuel.

Somehow, though, I fared forward. I jogged–shuffled toward the finish line, feeling the back side of my body crumple toward the ground like a paper accordion. Friends cheering near the finish line told me afterward I was a sickly shade of white and my face was locked in a ghastly grimace. Each time my heel hit the ground, the impact thundered up my body, crashing into waves of nausea. I struggled to keep my head up. Somewhere in the crowd of spectators stood 7-year-old Phoebe, and I didn't want her to see me falter and tumble to the ground.

Later, as Lynn and I started the drive back to Portland, we talked about those final 365+ yards of the race. Lynn complimented me, saying it takes a talented athlete to parcel out her energy so perfectly to have nothing left at the end. "How did you do it this time?" she asked, turning to look at me in the passenger seat.

Before I could answer, a torrent of tears, a mixture of happy and proud ones, poured forth. I didn't know being mentally tough could also mean being so emotional. My voice broke as I choked

PRACTICAL *Motherly* ADVICE
BUILDING MENTAL MUSCLE

Want to make your mind as strong as your quads? Follow my lead.

♀ Take no pity-prisoners. If you feel sorry for yourself while you run, you'll be miserable. You have chosen to run, so try to embrace the entire activity, aching knees and chub-rub included.

♀ Push a little farther with each workout. If you ran 10 miles, total, one week, go for 11 the next. If you generally avoid hills, tackle one instead of turning away. Go another 30 seconds on the treadmill at a faster pace than you did last week. Putting the bar just a little higher than you went last time builds your mental toughness as surely as it does aerobic capacity.

♀ Log your accomplishments. To shore up your mental reserves, remember the details of what you've done. Instead of simply jotting down miles, time, and maybe the course, note things like, "Ran up Trinity Pass hill with no walking breaks." Or, "Did reservoir loop solo after Laura was a no-show."

♀ Set small goals. On longer runs, for example, if you feel like you're hitting a wall, tell yourself if you plow through for 10 more minutes (or 1 more mile, or whatever goal makes sense), you can stop for water or walk or slow down for a minute. Breaking runs down into smaller segments makes them less daunting. As Lynn often told me, "Chunk it up."

♀ Enlist reinforcements. Having a running partner or group holds you accountable and keeps you on track. Supposed to go 10 miles this Sunday to prep for your first half-marathon? A friend by your side can make sure you do 10 instead of calling it quits at mile 8. When you start trying to run faster, a running partner can elicit healthy competition; nobody wants to be the first one to call "uncle." For better or worse, stubbornness paves the way to mental fortitude.

♀ Use visualization. Not in an "I can see myself winning" kind of way but in a far more simplistic way. I picture a place toward the end of my run here in Portland, like the intersection of Northeast 21st and Knott or the Vera Katz statue, and I imagine myself being there. Then I tell myself in very matter-of-fact terms, "Sarah, you are here now, but at some point in the future, you'll be there, so keep running."

9 Play the part. We're not elite athletes, but it doesn't mean we can't steal a few plays from their training manual. Doing drills like high knee lifts or skipping, which encourage rapid foot turnover, will make you feel and run like a pro.

9 "Reward" yourself after a double-digit run with an ice bath, which simultaneously builds character and minimizes soreness. My weekly ice bath kept me injury-free—and nearly devoid of any post-run soreness—while I trained for marathon #5. Take the plunge: Sit up to your waist in a tub of frigid water with a slew of ice floating in it for 10 to 15 minutes. (Stay warm by wearing a fleece jacket and wool hat. Distract yourself by reading a trashy magazine or playing with your iPhone, like I did.) Jump into a hot shower afterward to restore blood flow to your now-crimson legs.

out a reply, "Instead of retreating from the pain, I continued to move toward it." Then I chuckled, explaining that somewhere inside my fogged-up head, I'd heard the refrain, "Walk toward the light, Carol Ann. Walk toward the light."

In the summer after that race, I set two more personal bests, in 5K and 10K races. Sure, my times can be partly attributed to the speed I had developed through the workouts Lynn had me doing in the winter and spring. But more importantly, my brain was as coltish as my legs were. I didn't snap the finish tape at Eugene, but I busted through restraints I'd had in my head. I went from fighting the pain to embracing it. Instead of shying away from the lactic acid and the burning lungs, I now push toward them, knowing I can handle both capably. When a slice of my brain tells me to let up on the pace, a bigger part tells me to keep pressing on the accelerator.

It's as if pre-Eugene, when confronted with a line of pain, I would go up to it, and maybe peer over it to see what lay on the other side, but definitely not cross it. Post-Eugene, I now plow over it and get intimate with suffering. Because now I know, with certainty, I will survive. It might not be pretty—barfing and shaking muscles, anyone?—but the victorious feeling is beyond beautiful.

I don't mean to sound like a drill sergeant, but if your body never knows what it feels like to go longer, harder, or faster, your mind will never trust that it can. And the only way you can force your mind to believe is by crossing your own fence, too. You don't have to gun it for 26.2 miles, but you do have to push it for a set period of time. How long depends on your fitness level, but here's a guideline: Go long enough so you're super uncomfortable and every fiber of you is screaming at your brain to tell your body to slow down. Then go at least a minute—or 5—longer.

Run LIKE THIS MOTHER
MENTAL TOUGHNESS? CHECK.

By Dimity

I have a tough time with the concept of mental toughness. It has such a hard, metallic connotation, like I'm gunning to be one of the few, the proud, the Marines, which I'm definitely not. And it also feels like a chore: I have to run regularly, stretch, strength train, and cultivate mental toughness? I'll pass, thanks.

Conveniently for me, I don't think mental toughness needs to be built. Although I rationally know you have to accept pain in order to get better, I also believe this: As a runner, no matter your level or mileage, you are, by definition, mentally tough. There's a reason why less than 10 percent of this country runs, and why the elliptical machines and recumbent bikes fill up at the gym way before the treadmills do. Running isn't physically enjoyable. It takes discipline and courage to propel yourself forward faster than a walk. So whether you come in 5th or 5,000th in a race, realize you have more mental toughness than 99 percent of the people you've encountered in your life.

After two decades of running, I don't doubt I am mentally strong, but I also know I have zero interest in emptying my tank. I'm cool with that. For the most part, I step up to a challenge. To wit: My longest run before the Nike Women's Marathon was 16 miles, and I gritted out those last 3 while tearing up, wondering how I would be able to add 10.2 more, come race day, which was then a paltry 21 days away. Three weeks later (and a few more tears), I went the distance. The last 6 miles were a walk–jog–hobble, for which I make no apologies. That day, my needle rode in the red zone, and I was tougher than I've ever been.

I have a few things that substitute for having a steely brain. I'm anal, which works in my favor two ways: I hate not completing anything I've started, and I love crossing items off my to-do list. I'm also a classic middle child of divorced parents, so I crave praise, which I get after a race or tough workout, either from myself or from Grant, if I actually have a few uninterrupted minutes to tell him about it. I've found peer pressure elicits mental toughness as well; in a group setting or when I have to report my numbers back to a coach, I'm much more willing to push myself than when I'm solo. With respect to the Nike marathon? I wanted the cute T-shirt, the Tiffany necklace, and a magazine story that ended in glory, not dismay.

I don't really have a mantra to get me through the tough spots. I count my steps, or I set up really reachable goals (a tree 10 feet ahead, for instance), and I keep plodding along. The biggest mental challenge I ever set for myself was in a 10-mile race: During the first mile, I had to pass 10 people, the second mile, 9 people, the third, 8, and so on until I passed 1 during the last mile. I nailed it, and doing so kept my feet quick. Before that race and others, I remind myself of a line I've bastardized from a high-minded philosopher, which has stuck in my head for more than a decade: The body is able what the mind is willing.

Call mental toughness what you want. I say, when you call yourself a runner, you've already got the willing part down.

That experience, whether it's on the track, climbing hills, or doing interval work, retrains your mind along with your lungs. Suddenly, you'll realize burning isn't a bad thing; it's the desired outcome. Through those workouts you also learn you, too, will survive, you will recover, and you will run again, faster than last time because now you know you can. In a way, mental toughness is the opposite of childbirth: Moms say it's only after forgetting the torture of pushing out a baby that they can feel ready to get pregnant and give birth again. With running, it's holding onto the distinct memory of conquering pain that lets us do it all over again.

Don't shake your head and say some folks can do it, but you can't. Those exact same thoughts paraded around inside my head for days before the marathon. Even with Olympic coaching, I questioned whether I could pull it off. I looked for reassurances everywhere, asking every seasoned marathoner I knew, "How do you deal with the pain?" In their replies, they all sounded like masochists, saying the pain told them they were working hard. Instead of pushing through the hurt and trying to emerge on some mythical other side, they had trained themselves to be all right with the pain. They had accepted that to reach their goals, they had to run as close to empty as possible—and eventually, they'd get to their happy place, the finish line. I now know exactly what they're talking about, and I'm a better runner because of it.

I don't think I'll ever stop feeling limited by my tall, broad-shouldered, dimpled-in-places body, but I can continue honing my mind to be accepting, even welcoming, of pain. Because that light I'm running toward, I'm certain, is never going to dim.

.2 IF FAMOUS WOMEN WERE RUNNERS
By Sarah

How would the lives of famous females, either fictitious or real, be different if they'd laced up their sneaks and rubbed on the Bodyglide? History just wouldn't be the same.

IF EVE had been a runner, she would have swapped fig leaves for a sports bra.

IF CLEOPATRA had taken up running, she would've quickly learned sweat and kohl eyeliner don't mix. Instead, she would've used her natural beauty—and her killer legs—to woo lovers.

IF JULIET had been on her high school cross-country team, she never would have fallen so hopelessly in love with that Romeo fellow; being a harrier was a far more positive outlet for her youthful exuberance. Plus, her teammates would never have let her get so moony over a guy from another high school.

IF BETSY ROSS had been a runner, the American flag might be red with a block of blue with a few stars smattered on it. No time for sewing when there are Minuteman mile repeats to run.

IF JANE AUSTEN heroine Elizabeth Bennett had been a runner, she would have had the verdant grounds of Pemberley crisscrossed with running paths after finally marrying Mr. Darcy. (Although if he really looked like Colin Firth, she might never have left the estate's master bedroom!)

IF SACAGAWEA had been a runner, it would not have been called the Lewis and Clark Expedition. The fearless Shoshone woman would have led the whole way to the Pacific, with her infant son lashed to her back.

IF LOUISA MAY ALCOTT had been a trail runner, her semi-autobiographical classic about Meg, Jo, Beth, and Amy would certainly have been titled *Little Runners*, with a chapter about Jo racing next-door neighbor Laurie while her sisters cheered her on.

IF BETTY CROCKER had run as much as she baked, GU would've been invented in the 1940s, and the packets would've been filled with pure frosting.

IF AMELIA EARHART had been a running devotee, she would've jammed her running shoes into the cockpit so she could've taken a victory lap on the other side of the Atlantic.

IF EMILY POST had been a runner, she never would have worn earbuds in a race, fired off a snot-rocket—the horror!—or used a porta-potty. Or sweated, for that matter.

IF VIRGINIA WOOLF had run as well as she wrote, the endorphins would have helped pull her out of her depression. She would have run by the river instead of walking into it.

IF COCO CHANEL had done tempo runs down the Avenue des Champs-Élysées, running skirts would have become fashionable nearly a century ago.

04

CLOTHING: **DRESSING FOR SUCCESS**

By Dimity

As stereotypically girly as it sounds, I care about what I look like when I run. Anything above my neck doesn't matter so much—my hair is usually in the latest bed-head style, and face is often dotted with forgotten zit cream—but my clothes do. Not only do the right duds make the difference between comfortable and chafed, but I'm also confident there's some yet unproven scientific connection between clothes that look good and fast and feeling good and fast. I need every advantage I can get, so I pick wisely. Maybe one day, in my spare time, I'll apply for a grant from the National Science Foundation to get that study rolling, but in the meantime, here are some thoughts on the ultimate runner's wardrobe.

BRA

There's a woman whom I pass regularly on the bike path near my house. She's not a runner but a power walker, emphasis on the *power*—a real strider who thrusts up an arm with each gigantic step she takes. A good workout for sure, but I cringe every time I see her. She's well endowed—at least a D cup—and I'd generously put her odds at 50/50 that she's wearing a sports bra (or, actually, any bra). It certainly doesn't look like it. As she bounds along, her ta-tas, bouncing up and down, accumulate as much mileage as her feet do. I'm no scientist, but I do know this: After nursing two piglets, my boobs look like empty tube socks, so I can write with certainty that breast tissue is about as resilient as taffy. I can't imagine it's good to speed up her inevitable to-the-navel droop by slamming G-forces on her chest with every stride. Whenever I pass her, I say, "Hi," averting my eyes from the bobbing wreckage. What I'd like to plead is, "Please, come with me and get fitted for a bra. I'll even pay for it."

Run LIKE THIS MOTHER
A PLUG FOR ARTIFICIAL ENHANCEMENT

If my pink padded bra from Moving Comfort is clean, it's always my first choice. Although the additional endowment doesn't hurt the cause, what I like most is that it hides the headlights that inevitably flash into high beam when I'm cold or sweaty (read: pretty much whenever I run). After giving birth to children—and having a veritable parade prodding at my most private parts—I'm far from modest. But something about my covered nipples standing at attention makes me feel very exposed and self-conscious. I'd rather have you look me in my eyes, thanks.

Whether you're a DD or blessed with a meager B+ cup, like moi, those suckers can move when you're on the move. Think 10 × 800-meter repeats sound painful? Consider this: When you're running, breasts, no matter their size, can slam up and down 8 inches. Eight unbelievable, wince-inducing inches, which is the width of a piece of typing paper or, in more practical terms, the distance between your fingertips and the stuffed animal your child has dropped and has to have *right now*, even though you're piloting your minivan at 75 miles an hour. Ouch. And that's just one direction of movement; in 2007, researchers at the University of Portsmouth, England, found that breasts, as well-rounded as we imagine our children to be, also shimmy side to side and in and out.

Which is why I always tell new runners a dependable sports bra can be more critical than a good pair of running shoes. When you first try running and you circle your block a couple times, you can get by with wearing Converse tennies—if the *Chariots of Fire* folk did it, you can too—or Skechers, those pseudo-athletic shoes, and you probably will be no worse for the wear. But if you don't have the right bra, your first—and probably last—run will be miserable. Not only will you be physically uncomfortable, your cheeks may turn prematurely red. Most women I know, aforementioned strider excluded, don't want to draw attention to themselves, let alone their chest, as they sweat. If your ladies seem like they're waving to every passerby, chances are you're not going to give them another chance to be the welcoming committee.

So how to find your perfect bra? Trial and error. Or, rather, try-all and error. Start by getting measured, ideally by a knowledgeable woman on staff at a running or athletic apparel store, then scoop up as many appropriate bras as you can carry to the dressing room. Try a range of styles: pull-over-the-head, snap-in-back, zip-in-front, encapsulated cups, padded front. ("Zip in front?" you say, incredulously, "Never." *How do you know you don't like it if you haven't tried it?* echoes your mother in your head). Jog in place in front of the mirror and see how locked and loaded you are. Buy the ones that keep the ladies in line.

One warning: If you've never taken sports bra shopping seriously (read: you toss one in your cart at Target) you'll be in for some sticker shock. Most capable bras, for ladies with C cups and higher, can run at least $35 and often significantly more. (Those less endowed might be able to get away with bras from the Bull's-Eye Boutique.) I will make this promise, though: You'll never regret spending money on a bra that ensures your bust doesn't bust a move.

Shop LIKE THIS MOTHER
MY FAVES FOR . . .

BRAS: Title Nine stores and catalog, where bra fitting is taken as seriously and scientifically as NASA takes launching the space shuttle, and Moving Comfort, a company whose mission seems to be designing a style for every type from twiggy yogis to busty Athenas. (titlenine.com and movingcomfort.com)

PRE- AND POST-RACE WEAR: Running Divas, a company based in San Luis Obispo, California. They design stylish shirts with slyly sarcastic statements like "freakishly strong" and "high mileage" and "marathon mom" typed, in lowercase letters, across the chest. (runningdivas.com)

PANTS IN HARD-TO-FIND LENGTHS: Lucy and Athleta, two online and bricks-and-mortar retailers who peddle stylish women's sportswear, offer more styles in long and petite than I've ever seen. I can't praise them enough; I no longer look like I'm ready for any surprise river crossings that might suddenly pop up on my suburban, sidewalked routes. (lucy.com and athleta.gap.com)

PREGNANCY WEAR: Bornfit knows that although you'd like to look decent while sporting a beach ball on your stomach, comfort is the priority. Their bike shorts, skirts, shorts, tops, and lifestyle wear, all of which are designed for a ballooning belly, cover both bases. If you become addicted to their soft fabrics and flattering designs while pregnant, take heart: They also offer the same styles in regular sizes. (bornfit.com)

TANKS

The only thing truly small on my Amazonian frame is my chest. Which means I can wear tanks—the thick-strapped kind with a built-in shelf bra—without a second thought. (Despite a couple innovative models trying to change the mold, built-in bras in tanks generally aren't kind to larger-busted women, I'm sad to report.) On most days from spring to fall, it's my top of choice for a few reasons: It's easier to put on one tank than a bra and shirt; I tend to get hot quickly, and I feel coolest when my arms are exposed, but there's no way I'm baring my stretch-marked midsection wearing just a sports bra; I'm a slow runner, but my kids are veritable cinder blocks, so I have cut arms. (When do the "carry me?" whines end, by the way? By age 8, I'm hoping.) Their definition doesn't make up for my lack of foot speed, but at least runners who pass me feel speedy because I look stronger than I am.

Don't buy a super-tight tank or one made of thin seamless fabric; it'll just inch up as you run, which creates a muffin top even if you don't have one and, more importantly, is really annoying. Make sure it has at least one pocket to store small necessities; my massive minivan remote never fits in the doll-sized inner pockets in shorts. Some ingenious ones have a key pocket in the middle of your chest, where it definitely won't get lost.

One final note: Please save spaghetti-strap tanks for when your book group meets at a wine bar. Runners tend to be a forgiving crowd, fashion-wise, but dental floss straps don't give anybody in motion, save prepubescent 8-year-olds, the support they need or respect they deserve.

SHIRTS

How many times have you read, "Don't wear cotton when you run"? I agree with that sentiment in theory: Because it soaks up sweat, you risk hypothermia when it's freezing out and overheating when it's stifling out, blah blah blah. In reality, I love the occasional run in a super-soft, moisture-holding, pitted out cotton tee. I whittled my collection down to a few beloved tees, and when I want to feel like I've got nothing invested in a run, when I don't care how fast or hard or long I go, I throw one on and soak it. (This was a shocker for Sarah, a bit of a synthetic-fiber snob, who shudders every time she sees runners in natural materials.)

That said, those no-agenda runs usually are about 30 minutes long. If you're going longer, a top made of wicking fabric is definitely a better call: You'll stay drier when you run, and when you're done you'll avoid the chills. I own a few, but some inexplicable personality quirk makes me pretty averse to wearing technical T-shirts: I want my arms either totally covered or totally bare. Or maybe it's because I once wore a slightly small tech-tee in a race—I wore it because the shirt was red, and

TAKE IT *From* A MOTHER
WHAT'S YOUR FAVORITE PIECE OF RUNNING CLOTHING OR OUTFIT?

"My hot pink and black wicking yoga pants. I actually never owned anything pink before I started running, and now I can't get enough of it."

—KRISTYN (do you feel guilty when you run? no. "I come home feeling fabulous, and that feeling spreads to my family.")

"My uniform coat: Nike Dri-FIT, zip-up, black. Ancient. My mom has one and so does my running partner. I love it."

—KELLY (favorite feeling: after morning workout, spending the whole day on "runned" legs.)

"A Brooks skirt and singlet, with no bra. I'm flat when I'm not nursing, and I hate to have anything around my ribs/ chest when I exercise. I think it hinders my breathing."

—KAMI (signing up for a marathon soon? "A 5K sounds delicious, probably because I just gave birth.")

"My Sugoi red running shorts and The North Face tank top, because that means I'm running outside when it's warm and sunny."

—IVANA (favorite time to run: between 3 and 5 P.M. "My body is looser then.")

"My Brooks neon reflective jacket. I call it my 'I don't want to die' jacket."

—WENDY (best strength moves: squats and lunges.)

"My running skirt. There's something about feeling feminine when you know you look like hell."

—TINA (worst part of running: the first 20 minutes. "It takes me forever to get warmed up.")

the race was on the 4th of July—and ended up with an armpit rash so raw, I needed regular applications of A+D Diaper Ointment for more than a week to soothe it. (The tee was also brand new, which is an embarrassing rookie mistake made by a should've-known-better veteran. To avoid emptying your kid's stash of diaper rash cream unnecessarily, be sure to wear your competition garb at least twice on runs at least two thirds as long as your race.)

PRACTICAL *Motherly* ADVICE
YOU'RE GOING OUT IN THAT?

Given that you probably have assembled at least 10,000 outfits in your lifetime, we're not going to dole out the Garanimals approach to dressing. But here are a few things to consider when suiting up:

- Fall through spring, dress like it's 10 degrees warmer outside than it really is. You'll be chilly initially but will heat up quickly. If you're not shivering a bit while standing around outside, waiting for a friend to show up, shed a layer before you head out.

- Summertime, look for loose-fitting tops with tightly woven fabrics. (If you hold it up to a light, the less light that shines through, the better.) Also, opt for darker colors, which absorb UV rays, unlike lighter colors, which let the rays pass through.

- Save ugly, overlogo'ed race tees for marathons, which usually start at the cold crack of dawn. Wear it for a few miles, then toss it on the sidewalk. (Many of the larger marathons gather up the discarded clothes and donate them.)

- Compression wear—tights, socks, and tops with tightly woven fabric to shunt oxygen-rich, healing blood to tired muscles—is becoming more widespread. Tri-geeks and speedier runners are adopting them for races, resulting in a modified "Hot for Teacher" sort of look. Runners usually use them for recovery after a tough workout or during long plane trips, when blood flow to the legs can be compromised. If you're going for a PR and are flying from, say, San Diego to Boston, you might consider forking over $100 for a pair of tights to wear on the plane and after the marathon. Otherwise, I'd advise to save your cash (and if you're flying, get up frequently and walk the aisle).

VESTS

Sarah and I are yin and yang about vests: She loves them, I hate them. I think, "What's the point? Either commit with arms or get out." She, on the other hand, reveres them. They protect her from light rain—or "liquid sunshine," as Portlanders lovingly call it—and she thinks they offer just the right amount of warmth for temps in the low 50s, a common spot on the thermometer in her hometown. Plus, she's addicted to her Nikeplus iPod, and a vest, unlike a long-sleeve tee, offers pockets for stashing it, plus a gel or two.

JACKETS

A lightweight jacket is a good basic to have in your repertoire: It's ammunition you can use to shoot down the excuse, "It's too cold or rainy to run." Key things you want: a pocket or two, a few hits of reflectivity, and a water-resistant classification. (Don't wear something that's totally waterproof: You'll end up steamier than the latest Nora Roberts novel.)

Since Sarah and I peel off our jackets about as frequently as Sarah's twins stripped naked as toddlers, we've had plenty of opps to figure out the best way to knot a jacket. The best is the twist-and-roll: Holding an arm of shed jacket in each hand, twist the sleeves in opposite directions, like you're rolling a towel to snap somebody. The body of the jacket coils around the arms and turns into a long fabric tube. Then tie it around your waist, thus avoiding any unflattering bulge or annoying flap.

UNDIES

When it comes to exercising, I'm the female equivalent of Free Willy. I don't like panty lines under my yoga pants; I fundamentally don't understand thongs, which avoid said lines; I think running shorts are lined for a reason. For the sake of your girl-bits, I hope most of you are with me on this one, at least when it comes to running. (I've seen plenty of panty lines as I glance around—not inward, as I should be—in yoga, so I realize I could be in the minority there.) But it doesn't take an OB/GYN to figure out sweating in heat- and moisture-trapping cotton undies under a wicking liner isn't a good call. Unless, of course, you like to end your run at Walgreen's to stock up on yeast-fighting Vagisil.

LYCRA SHORTS

The linked-sausage look that tight-fitting compression shorts bring to your legs isn't the most flattering, especially when they're worn by middle-aged male marathoners, who seem to favor pulling them down to their knees. But when the alternative is red, angry thigh chafe, I'll take the linked look any day. I wore them constantly in the late '90s, but now I often wear shorts designed for trail running or a running skirt, both of which have a built-in longer liner, on epic training runs.

SHORTS

Amazingly enough, I'm not super picky about running shorts. I favor darker colors—blacks and grays, which match with anything, hide spills, and de-emphasize my child-bearing hips—and prefer fabrics to be medium weight. Featherweight, paper-thin shorts, though good in theory, tend to get weighed down by keys or gels, and suddenly I'm baring serious crack, a look I'm not fond of. I like the inseams to be 3 inches or so; longer than that ages me prematurely, and shorter makes me look like a mom who is trying too hard to hold onto her glory days.

In fact, shorts with an inseam less than 2 inches, including bun huggers, should be worn only if you're on a high school track team or you're a woman with 13 percent body fat who regularly wins races. Why? They're the athletic equivalent of a pair of Abercrombie's low-slung jeans. The jeans reveal too much of the top of your bum, and the running shorts let the bottom half of it hang out. Either way, it's too much information.

And since I'm dispensing my valuable fashion wisdom, here's another tidbit. It takes a very special (read: very fit, very confident, very taut) runner to pull off the classic split-leg running shorts, the ones with peek-a-boo slits up both sides. After all, they're designed to showcase your wheels with every long, perfectly executed stride. Proceed with caution.

Even if you've got glutes you can display proudly in windy situations, under no circumstances should your shorts resemble a flag design. Wear your patriotism (or your Texas pride) somewhere other than on your ass, please.

RUNNING SKIRTS

When skirts first burst onto the scene, they seemed just a tad less divisive than the death penalty. You either loved the feminine look or hated it. But slowly, like platform heels, skinny jeans, and any other fashion that initially seems ridiculous but later trickles down to Old Navy, skirts have become popular enough that you don't look twice at a runner flitting down the path in one.

Skirts get a hearty two thumbs up from this crowd, a pair who aren't especially known for being feminine and flirty. First off, as mentioned before, most skirts have a decently long liner, which keeps your thighs from gnashing at each other angrily. Second, a skirt doesn't restrict range of motion, so you can gallop down hills and not worry about splitting any seams. Third, there's no better pick for a race pic. Running shorts can often bunch up in between the legs, creating an unsightly bulge in the front most race photographers seem to have a gift for capturing. Finally, when I'm wearing a skirt, it's hard to take myself too seriously. I love how I can feel it swishing along, like it's enjoying the ride as much as I am.

Some people will never be skirt wearers, and others, like Sarah, will never go back. I'm about 50/50 skirts and shorts; I tend to train in both but race in skirts. I find there's an understood connection when you see another skirt at a race. It makes me feel like part of an unspoken team.

If you're feeling self-conscious about wearing one, try it out at a female-dominant race, like a Race for the Cure or SkirtChaser 5K, where you get a cute skirt, instead of getting a T-shirt, for entry. (Keep it under 10K if the skirt is brand new so you don't make the same T-shirt mistake I did.) I went all out when we ran the Nike Marathon, wearing a black running dress from SkirtSports. I got more compliments than I expected and never once doubted my choice, which kept me chafe-free and cool the entire time. That said, if the race were co-ed, I wouldn't have been so bold.

TIGHTS

There seems to be a direct relationship between the seriousness of the runner and the cliginess of her Lycra on her lower half. Yoga pants say, "I'm a casual runner, and I don't mind if I trip on these bell bottoms, since I'll iron out my muscular kinks later in the studio." Loose tights, the kind with zippers on the bottom that your 4th-grade gym teacher used to wear, say, "I'm getting faster, but my quads are not quite honed enough for a 3-D display." (Or, "I secretly wanted to be a P.E. teacher.") And those no-room-for-error tights, worn without tied-around-the-waist butt coverage? They scream, "Make no mistake, sister. These (single-digit body fat) legs were made for running."

Running through Minnesota winters and various body weights, I've worn all three styles, and they all work well. But these days, I'm over long pants for running. I simply don't like them anymore. With the exception of yoga pants, I feel like they make me look too serious, and I hate how they make my feet look like water skis protruding out from their tapered ankles.

My semi-perfect solution, now that I live in milder Colorado, where winter temps tend to range between 35 and 50 degrees, is capris. They lend the same casual sassiness to my style as a skirt does, but they are also practical. They banish chafe and give the knee and its ligaments a bit of extra support. If it's below 35, I'm usually in my yoga pants (or inside, on the treadmill).

Sarah also bares half her legs in cooler temps, braving even colder temps in capris than I do. Marathon training during a chilly spring had her doing all her long runs in capris, making her realize she missed chub-rub about as much as 2 A.M. breastfeeding sessions. Even though her marathon was in early May and it ended up being about 58 degrees, Sarah raced in her capris. Her quads might have felt like cement blocks by the end, but at least she didn't feel like sandpaper was rubbing her thighs raw along the way.

.2   T-SHIRT SLOGANS WE LOVE

"I'm the fast woman your mother warned you about."

"Why couldn't Pheidippides have dropped dead at the 20-mile mark?"

"This seemed like a good idea 3 months ago!" (spotted during a marathon)

"Hard things take time to do. Impossible things take a little longer."

"If you think this is hard, try chemotherapy." (worn by a Team in Training member)

"In my dreams, I'm Kenyan."

"Does this shirt make my ass look fast?"

Front: "No, I don't do steroids." Back: "But thanks for asking."

Front: "Half-marathon ready." Back: "At all times."

"If found on ground, please drag across finish line."

"Runs when chased." (made by a daughter for her dad)

"Find your happy pace."

"All it takes is all you have."

"I will keep running until I no longer feel beautiful doing it."

05

SHOES: CHATTING WITH YOUR SOLEMATES

By Sarah

As Sarah Jessica Parker made so abundantly and brilliantly clear in *Sex and the City*, we women love our shoes. We shop our way out of depression in the Nordstrom shoe department. We spend small fortunes on Christian Louboutins and Manolo Blahniks. (Or at least Sarah Jessica does. I spend meager amounts on Clarks and Kenneth Coles.) Yet as runners we ought to be paying more attention to—and possibly spending more money on—our running shoes, not the black boots we wear to the office or the silvery ballet flats we wear on date night. (How many hubbies actually notice anything we're wearing below the waist, anyway?)

Why? We are more intimate with our running shoes than with any other pair in our closets. They support us through miles and miles. They know weaknesses about us we might not even be aware of. They absorb our stink and our sweat. They let us wear them down.

And for all the abuse we give them, they barely even bat a shoelace. (OK, maybe they let out a squeak once in a while.) In the interest of fairness, we're giving our most devoted pair of shoes the chance to speak their minds in this chapter. Just short rants, though; we already field way too many complaints from things below eye level.

"ARE YOU SURE WE'RE RIGHT FOR EACH OTHER?"

Staring down a wall of running shoes can be as daunting as being faced by all the guys at a freshman mixer. So many choices. Which boy will hold you close—but not too close—as you sway to a Whitney Houston hit? Or, translated out of high school angst, which shoe will cradle your heel, hug your arch, and give your toes room to spread as you tromp along? Take the guesswork out of it and put your feet in the hands of a salesperson at a running specialty store, the equivalent of the gossipy friend in ninth grade who knew that Scott, not Todd, had a crush on you.

If you're a beginning runner, just going into a running specialty store can be intimidating. Look in the window, and you're likely to see a scrawny staffer with 5 percent body fat who thinks running 70 miles in 7 days qualifies as a recovery week. Two things to know about hardcore runners, though: They're passionate about getting other people running, and they're also total geeks about running gear. What's more, you're definitely not the first possibly not-so-in-shape person to walk in, cop to the fact you're a beginner or beginning again, and have no clue about shoes. So once you get up the courage to head in and explain your situation, Mr. Chiseled-Calves will happily check out your running style—sometimes on a treadmill, sometimes on the sidewalk—and suggest shoes based on how your foot hits the ground and what it does as you roll through your stride. Feel free to ask lots of questions; Mr. C.-C. loves spewing running knowledge. Then he'll suggest several different brands at a range of prices, so you will still have the final call. No arranged marriages here.

"DON'T CHEAT YOURSELF."

Don't settle on a pair of cheap running shoes; they're the equivalent of sleeping on a rock-hard futon. Yes, it works for a night, but a week into it, your bones feel downright geriatric. If you run more than 4 or 5 miles a week, you deserve better. When you shortchange your feet, you are flirting with pain and injury, including sore knees and shin splints. Running shoe prices, which broke the three-digit barrier several years ago, continue to climb, but you can still get an excellent pair for $85–$95. (No cheap date, to be sure, but remember: Shoes are really the only piece of equipment you need for our beloved sport.) Spend more—$110 and up—and you get a higher grade of materials and technology, which some runners think is worth the money. Decide for yourself, but for the sake of your body, skip the $30 kicks at Payless or Wal-Mart.

"LOOK INTO MY SOLE FOR ANSWERS."

The bottom part of your current running shoes can tell you so much about what your feet do when you run and thus what you should look for in your next pair of sneaks. Namely, they can tell if you overpronate or if you have a neutral stride.

Greek to you? You might have heard the term *overpronator* bandied about by Mr. C.-C. and his gaunt tribe. That $5 word gets applied when a runner's foot turns inward (toward the arch) too much after hitting the ground. Compare that to the term *neutral*. No, not a runner who looks good in beige but one whose foot doesn't roll over excessively. (Everyone's foot pronates to some degree because it's

Run LIKE THIS MOTHER
CUSTOM ORTHOTICS: SAVIOR OR STUPID?

By Dimity

In the past two decades, I've had three pairs of custom orthotics made for my problematic feet. My first pair, a three-quarter-length style, came in high school, after a podiatrist spied how high my arches were; my second, full-length pair came in college; and my final pair, also the full enchilada, entered my life (and my shoes) about 2 years ago, to prevent another stress fracture in my heel. In between pairs, I used off-the-rack insoles from Sole, which seemed costly at $40 a pop, but considering that custom orthotics cost $300 or more, they were a bargain. The Soles felt very supportive; I completed the training for two half-Ironman triathlons in them with no problems, save exhaustion.

I know some people swear by their custom orthotics, and I wish I could too. But I honestly don't know if any pair really made a difference in preventing injuries or creating a more efficient running stride. Although it felt good to have a mold under my foot that cradled it perfectly, they also felt so aggressive—my most recent pair felt like I had golf balls under my arches—I worried they didn't allow the relaxed, natural movement my injury-prone lower body wanted. In fact, one of the first days of wearing my most recent pair, I severely twisted my ankle while slowly walking down the stairs; my hunch is the ligaments and tendons in my foot were being held in place so rigidly, they couldn't self-correct.

When a super-knowledgeable running gait specialist suggested I ditch my last pair, I happily complied. Then I asked him what I should've done differently. My biggest mistake: getting a pair made without a physical therapist or sports doctor looking at my running stride. Qualified experts customize orthotics much more accurately when they take your whole package—foot problems, running style, other injuries—into account, not just looking at your feet. All three of my pairs were just molded right from the doctors' chairs, with no questions about or illustrations of my running.

So here's my hard-won, expensive advice: If somebody suggests you need orthotics, ask about off-the-rack options first. Try those, and if they don't solve the problem, get another medical opinion. Chat up ol' Mr. C.-C. at the running shoe store and ask him for recommendations of podiatrists or orthopedists. Then be sure they see you in motion before you swipe your credit card.

TAKE IT *From* A MOTHER
WHEN DO YOU KNOW IT'S TIME FOR A NEW PAIR OF KICKS?

"I use coolrunning.com. When you enter in your mileage for the day, you can set up a sneakers category and track a pair's mileage. I also know it's time for a change when I start feeling soreness in my shins."

—DEBBIE (longest run: 27.2 miles. "One-mile warmup before the marathon.")

"I try to purchase new running shoes around a significant date or holiday so it's easier to remember the date of purchase."

—KELLY (first two marathons were in Ironman triathlons. "Third was when my fourth baby was 7.5 months old. My mom wanted to qualify for Boston, and I wanted to help her.")

"I use the online log at runningahead.com. I am pretty religious about tracking my mileage, but I don't replace shoes when I hit a certain number. Instead, I rotate a new pair of shoes around 250 miles. When I start getting minor plantar fasciitis, it's time to retire my older pair."

—RAQUEL (favorite race: Escape from Alcatraz Triathlon in 2008. "I saw it on TV when I was a kid and thought, 'One day, I'm going to do that.'")

"I look at the tread on the shoes and pay attention to whether they're losing their padding. I definitely don't keep track of the mileage. Who has time for that?"

—ROBYN (best part of running: feeling free. "As a mom, the only time the kid burden lightens is when I'm running or after they're in bed.")

the body's natural cushioning mechanism. Exercise Physiology 101: When a runner's foot hits the ground with up to three times the force of a walking stride, it needs to roll to some degree to absorb the extra impact.) There are also runners who supinate, or have their feet roll outward, but they are less than 5 percent of the crowd and should generally wear the same shoes as a neutral runner.

To figure out which camp you fall into, grab a pair of shoes with some miles on them. If the inside part of the sole at the heel is looking pretty thrashed, then count yourself part of the approximately 65 percent of runners who overpronate to some degree. (Or if you put your shoes on a table, look at them from the back. If they lean in toward each other, it's a sure sign you're an overpronator.) If the backside of your shoe is worn down fairly evenly, then you have a neutral stride.

Another way to tell? Take the wet test, a favorite among the crowd over at *Runner's World* magazine. Forget stepping on a piece of paper, as they always suggest—way too high maintenance. Just take a look the next time you step out of the shower onto the bathmat. If you can see pretty much all of the bottom of your foot or at least half of the middle part of your foot joining your heel and forefoot, then you have low to normal arches and are an overpronator. But if the wet mark joining the front and back of your foot is a sliver, it means you have a high arch and thus a neutral stride.

And all this means what? It determines whether you are better off in a cushioning, stability, or motion control shoe. Although all running shoes have cushioning, some also have plastic gizmos or extra-firm material on the inside of the heel to slow down foot roll for overpronators. If a shoe has some, but not a ton, of that kind of stuff, then it's called a stability shoe. If it has enough restraints to keep a juvenile delinquent in line, then it's called a motion control shoe. Neutral runners don't need all that extra stuff; they should just leave well enough alone and pick out a cushioning shoe. Confused? Mr. C.-C. will help. We promise. (*Love* him!)

"LOOKS CAN BE DECEIVING."

I'll forgive you if you just skimmed all my blah blah blah about pronation control this and cushioning that, if you promise me this: You won't buy your next pair of shoes based solely on appearances. I love light blue as much as the next gal, maybe even more, but when the update of my favorite running shoes came only with red accents, that's what I laced up. Matching be damned: How a shoe performs is what's important, not what it looks like. Like nursing bras, minivans, and other practical items we've resigned ourselves to accepting as mothers, running shoes are all about function.

"DON'T DRAG OUT OUR RELATIONSHIP."

Experts recommend getting a new pair of running shoes after 300 to 500 miles, which isn't that complicated to calculate, but does feel tedious to keep track of. So if you run 20 miles a week, they're cooked in about 3.5 to 6 months. (Create a cheat sheet by writing the date you debuted them on one tongue with the Sharpie floating around your kitchen.) Heavier runners should be on the shorter end of the range, lighter ones on the longer. Runners who store shoes in the sauna-hot trunk of a car or near a heating vent should also replace them sooner because heat speeds up the breakdown of rubber and cushioning materials. If you wear your running shoes to tool around in town (tsk, tsk!), make sure you factor that into your mileage tally. As you near the expiration date of a pair, buy a new pair and rotate between the two until the older pair feels flat and dead. Then you can wear *that* pair around town, and I won't judge you.

PRACTICAL *Motherly* ADVICE
TRAIL RUNNING SHOES: WORTH IT?

If you're an occasional trail runner or one who sticks to fairly well-worn paths that don't invoke the word *gnarly*, you'll be fine with your regular kicks (that is, if you're fine with your shoes being more gray than white when you're done). But you might want to spend $80 or so for a pair of trail runners if

- You run more on the trails than on the road. Most trail runners have a beefier midsole and an aggressive sole to provide underfoot protection and superior traction.

- You tackle trails that are pretty rocky and rooted or have tricky hills. Your feet won't get so beat up, and you'll feel more mountain goat-y.

- You hike a lot. We wear trail runners on long day hikes because they're lighter than boots or more sturdy hikers but feel just as capable.

- You run on snowshoes. Low-profile trail runners often fit the bindings of running-style snowshoes best.

"I THINK WE NEED SOME SPACE."

Seems a lot of us take after Cinderella's stepsisters, trying to cram our tootsies into shoes that are too small for us. Some studies have shown that as many as four out of five runners wear shoes at least a half size too short. To give your feet room to spread and move—and to prevent unsightly black toenails—you need to leave about a thumbnail's width of space between the end of your longest toe and the tip of your shoe. Some trail-trotters leave even more space in their trail shoes because feet tend to move around more on uneven surfaces. Pretend Mr. C.-C. is Prince Charming, and put him to work: Be sure to try on both left and right shoes at the store, because most folks have one foot that's slightly longer than the other. Shop for shoes at the end of the day, when your feet are at their most swollen, and wear your regular running socks.

"LET'S TIE THE KNOT."

Two words: Double knot.

"I FEEL LIKE YOU'RE SLIPPING AWAY FROM ME."

Women may come in all shapes and sizes, but our feet are often the same general shape: wide around the ball of the foot and narrow at the heel. As a result, our heels can slip up and down annoyingly in our shoes as we run, which is a surefire blister builder.

Instead of getting shoes that are narrower, adjust the way you lace your shoes. Start out the normal way, but after going through the next-to-last eyelet, pass each lace through the top eyelet on the same side, with the lace on top of the shoe material. This gives you a small loop. Now, put the ends of the laces through the opposite loops, give a good tug on the laces, and tie your shoes the regular way. Your heel should now feel more secure than a swaddled newborn.

"LOVE STINKS."

If the odor coming out of your shoes rivals the smell that hits you when you open a jar of minced garlic—tell me you don't actually chop individual cloves, do you?—take out the sock liner, then machine wash both the liners and the shoes in cold water on the gentle cycle. Either liquid or powder detergent works, but to minimize breakdown of the cushioning, don't machine wash your shoes more than once every 3 months. Then stuff 'em with newspaper and let both liners and shoes air dry overnight. Keep your kicks morning-breeze fresh by removing the sock liners after every run. If that doesn't help keep the stench at bay, sprinkle baking soda or baby powder in your shoes as well.

"LET'S TAKE A BREATHER."

If you're consistently logging 25 or more miles a week, consider having two pairs of running shoes and alternating them. The switch gives the cushioning materials time to rebound and the uppers and insoles to dry. Having two pairs of running shoes sounds like a splurge, but how many pairs of heels do you have? Boots? Flip-flops? Shoes you've worn once or never? We thought so. For a half-marathon or marathon, break in a new pair of shoes you'll race in by rotating them into your regular runs. Aim to have about 30 miles in your new shoes before race day so you'll know they're problem-free.

.2   SONGS WE WON'T ADMIT—UNTIL NOW—THAT WE LISTEN TO

As Jimmy Buffett's "Cheeseburger in Paradise" often reminds us, there are certain songs that are cool to belt out when you're drunk in college ("I like mine with lettuce and tomato, Heinz 57, and French-fried potato!") but should not ever be listened to sober. This admittedly corny playlist is in that embarrassing genre. We love it when they pop up in our rotations, but we're smart enough to keep our mouths shut while we listen. Most of the time, anyway. Sometimes, though, we have to proclaim, "I believe it's time for me to fly!"

"MMMBop" by Hanson

"Never Gonna Give You Up" by Rick Astley

"Hot Stuff" by Donna Summer

"Something About You" by Level 42

"Time for Me to Fly" by REO Speedwagon

"Pour Some Sugar on Me" by Def Leppard

"Wake Me Up Before You Go Go" by Wham!

"On the Road Again" by Willie Nelson

"Who Let the Dogs Out?" by Baha Men

"Centerfold" by the J. Geils Band

"I Would Do Anything for Love (But I Won't Do That)" by Meat Loaf

"Cracklin' Rosie" by Neil Diamond

"Jive Talkin'" by the Bee Gees

"Smooth Criminal" by Michael Jackson

"Flashdance: What a Feeling" by Irene Cara

"The Best" by Tina Turner

"Don't Stop Believin'" by Journey

"Believe" by Cher

"Macho Man" by The Village People

"Gimme Gimme Gimme" by Erasure

06

ACCESSORIES: GADGETS, GIZMOS, AND OTHER GOTTA-HAVES

By Dimity

Name a body part—head, waist, chest, wrists, fingers, eyes, feet—and you can cover it, strap something around it, or otherwise accessorize it for running. The options are enough to make a shopaholic trade a trip to the mall for a running store excursion. Almost. Because—and hopefully this isn't news to you—buying a water bottle holder, which looks suspiciously like a fanny pack, doesn't bring on quite the same rush as finding a Bottega Veneta purse that makes you feel chic and sophisticated. A water bottle holder will never make you feel cool.

But water will *keep* you cool when you're running; if there's ever a reason to embrace the mantra "function over fashion," running accessories are it. Stylish running clothes, about a decade overdue, are no longer an oxymoron, but accessories still trend toward clunky, nondescript, and unisex. They do serve their purpose, though: keeping you warm, hydrated, on track, entertained, whatever they're built to do. Which is to say, at mile 7, which you know is mile 7 because your watch just beeped to tell you so, you're still happily chugging along, hydrated because of your dorky water bottle holder, chafe-free because you're lubed up with Bodyglide, and comfortable because your socks are cushioned.

Despite the many advertised benefits on hangtags, there's no need to overaccessorize while running. Here, with a discerning eye, I'll run down what you need and why you need it.

SOCKS

I admit I have sticker shock often—a three-digit price tag on a pair of jeans still seems ridiculous to me, as does a latte that costs more than a worker in a third-world country makes in a week—but when I recently saw running socks retailing for $20 and up, I was astounded. Really? I mean, I know they're engineered down to the cubic millimeter to ergonomically cradle your arch, cushion your sole, and fit your left and right foot down to the toenails. Still, spending the equivalent of two movie tickets for a single pair of socks doesn't jibe for me.

Which isn't to say I buy a twelve-pack of cotton socks for $6.99 from Costco. Cotton socks, which turn mushy with sweat and dry out only when removed, bring on blisters faster than a rake handle on office-worker palms in autumn. There is a middle ground—somewhere in the $10 to $12 range—where intelligently designed running socks and my stinginess collide. I can stomach the price because the fabrics are sweat-wicking wool or polyester, the cushioning stays plush wash after wash, and the sock feels like ambrosia when you first put it on. As you should with shoes, find a style and brand that work well with your feet, and stick with them. (Plus, doing so makes it easier to make pairs when the devilish dryer eats one.)

I have a handful of favorite pairs, always in the front of my drawer, that are finally on their last leg. I like a thinner sock for the same reason I like scoop-neck tees: They just feel right on my body. Some have an *L* and *R* on the toes, but I usually get it wrong in my groggy early morning state, and I gotta say, I can't feel a difference when they're on the correct foot. (I'm a size 12 clodhopper, though, so I'm pretty sure I don't conform to the creative vision of most sock designers.) Some my big toe has poked through the end; others are so grungy, they look like they came out of a sewer, not a washing machine. They've still got plenty of miles left, though. By the time I'm finally willing to part with them, I'm sure they'll cost a few more dollars to replace.

ELECTRONIC GADGETS

If you're a true runner, you'll want something to keep track of most of your outings. (If you think *no, I really don't,* then chances are you're a yogini moonlighting as a runner.) The gadget can be your Swatch from junior year of high school or a geeky $400 GPS system that logs every nanostep you take, but having some way to track your pace—and tangibly see it improve—can be the difference between soldiering on or quitting. How? After a month of running, a newbie might notice she hits a certain mailbox 12 minutes into her route, not 14, as it used to be. Then, 2 months later, she pushes herself to reach it in 10 and becomes slightly obsessive about reaching that goal. She's become a runner. Or, thanks to her new gadget, a 9:30-mile runner suddenly realizes she's actually a 9:10 runner, and, lo and behold, she's ready to aim for a sub-9:00 pace for a half-marathon, something she never would've thought possible back in her 11-minute-mile days.

That kind of progress seems superficial in print, but it's surprisingly fulfilling in person. Even lacking most competitive genes, I thrive on feedback from my runs, even the embarrassingly slow ones. The numbers on my wrist testify to the work I've done, the miles I've covered, the time I've

(DON'T) *Run* LIKE THIS MOTHER
A KEY TO KEEPING YOUR KEYS SAFE

Where to stash your keys during a run is a problem without a solid solution: Inner pockets on shorts can be flimsy, sliding it between your girls invites chest-chafe, and zipping them into a jacket pocket creates a jangle that becomes increasingly annoying with every step. But all those options are better than the one my friend Amy, a mother of two daughters, previously used: tying it into her shoelace. I'll let her tell the story.

"I was running with a friend on Valentine's Day. It had recently snowed, and the trail was muddy. I had the master key to my car tied into my shoelace, but it must have been in the double-knot part, not the initial knot. I would've felt it if my shoe totally untied. Anyway, after running 9 miles, I realized that my key was gone. So we ran the whole trail again. It's hard to run and look straight at the ground (and through weeds, mud, and snow). No luck. My husband, much to his dismay, had to load up the kids and drive 30 miles to give me the only key we had left: the valet key.

"The next day, I took that key to Home Depot to get it copied, imagining it was an easy task. Ha. They don't copy valet keys. So I called the dealership, and they told me I had to get the whole car 'rechipped,' which would cost about $3,000. Not kidding. So I ran the trail one more time, looking for it, but still, no key.

"The good news is I got a new car out of the whole thing. My transmission was getting close to going out, so we just figured it was cheaper to put the money into a new car than sink an unexpected three grand into the old one."

Amy's moral of the story: Never take your key with you. She now has a handy hiding spot above her back tire that she uses.

Dimity's better moral: Lose a key, get a new car.

committed. These days, when much of the work I do goes undocumented and unappreciated, those numbers give my pride enough momentum to keep rolling through the days and miles.

SPORTS WATCH

A waterproof sports watch is a great call for a beginner: It's simple, not a huge investment, and holds up to everyday use, especially when you wash your poop- and snot-wiping hands more times than a nurse. I only use the basic stopwatch function—push "start" when you go, "stop" when you're done—and calculate any intervals I may be running in my head. I hate to read manuals, and even if I did, I can never find enough time to program something and then become fluent in it.

I do like to time my own races, though. Even if the race is chip timed (translation: a small gadget on your shoelaces or ankle records your time when you step on special mats at the start, along the way, and at the finish line), I'm still a DIY timer. Why? This may come as a surprise, but I don't line up in the front with the runners whose legs are roughly the diameter of my arms. Instead, I cross the starting line at least 45 seconds after the gun goes off, which gives me a nice, albeit false feeling of speediness when the race also displays splits along the course. "That clock reads 16:18, but I'm actually only at 14:58," I'll tell myself, feeling like I hold a secret nobody else has. For some reason, the longer the race, the bigger I build my imaginary cushion to be: A 90-second cushion turns into a 4-minute pillow by mile 10, which I pretend is a 10-minute bonus at mile 23. Reality hits when I cross the finish line, but by then I'm so relieved to be done, I don't really care.

HEART RATE MONITOR

Back in the early '90s, heart rate monitors, a combo watch and strap worn around your chest, were the next new thing: You could watch, beat by beat, how hard your heart was working as you ticked off the miles. I wore one fairly regularly, but I never really used it. As a fitness writer, although I'm well aware of heart rate zones and the reason for their existence, I learned quickly that heeding them is like trying to thread a needle on a treadmill. Impossible. So the number turned into more of a fascinating distraction than helpful information: *Look, I'm at 175 on the flats! I'm close to blowing up!* Or, *Wow: 134! I'm so fit! Actually, it might be I'm running downhill.*

Still, during cooldown walks, I liked to relive my runs via my monitor, which, as they became more advanced, spewed out average and max heart rates and—my favorite—calories burned. (*That run was seven Oreos! Score!*) But did I ever use those numbers while running to stay in my (never determined) correct aerobic zone or most efficient interval zone? No. Did I ever do anything with that information after my run? No.

Which is why my heart rate monitor is now semi-retired. After I hired a coach, who gave me zones and guidelines, I appreciated the monitor, and she used its data much more. But it was too little, too late: By then, gadgets that track pace had become the next new thing. Still, I keep my Polar monitor in my gym bag for times when I'm stuck indoors. Polar is the brand that is usually compatible with treadmills, ellipticals, stationary bikes, and other cardio equipment. I don't know about you, but I hate putting my sweaty hands on those electrode things, and Lord knows, I can't do an indoor workout without as much data as possible to distract me.

TAKE IT *From* A MOTHER
WHAT'S YOUR FAVORITE PIECE OF GEAR?

"My prescription Rudy Project sunglasses."

—CHARITY (runs early. "I used to be a pastry chef, and my day began at 5 A.M. I'm still ready to roll at 4:45.")

"Nike Free running shoes. I'm convinced they've made my feet stronger. They've eliminated my need for orthotics."

—ROBYN (do most of your friends get your running? "Probably not.")

"My hat! I hate having hair blowing in my face and sweat rolling down my face. The hat is essential!"

—REBA (do you keep track of race times? "Yes. Doesn't everybody?")

"Custom orthotics."

—STEPHANIE (favorite cross-training: Pilates. "Makes me feel skinny no matter how big the muffin top.")

"My Garmin. I'm anal about pace and distances."

—CARMEN (dream running date: fellow cancer survivor Lance Armstrong.)

"Balega socks. They're made in South Africa and worth every penny."

—MARY (dream race: Antarctic Marathon.)

GPS UNITS

I know, I make myself sound all chillaxed about splits, beats, and paces. Then I bought a Garmin Forerunner 305, a device that uses orbiting satellites to accurately and instantly track every step you take, and I became borderline OCD. Providing pace, time run, calories burned, distance covered, and probably some other stats I haven't yet discovered, GPS units are the digital cameras of the running world: You know quickly if you're looking good or should reconsider capturing this moment.

On my first 5.27-mile run with my Garmin, I must have looked at it roughly 250 times. Pace is so much more meaningful and tangible than heart rate that when I wear it, I can't just run anymore. I see a 10:13 pace on it and think, *Come on: You're faster than that, Dimity!* Four steps later, I'm at 7:30 and think, *OK, speedy, who do you think you are, Paula Radcliffe?* Four more steps, I'm at 8:40 and

Run LIKE THIS MOTHER
SWEET WHISPERS IN MY EAR

By Sarah

Although I usually run solo, at any point during my runs, I can hear a friendly voice in my ear. My omnipresent, imaginary running companion, whom I envision as a petite brunette with a sleek ponytail and quick smile, sometimes tells me how long I've been running. Other days she clicks off each mile I cover. At the end of every run, she's right there to tell my total run stats: time, distance, and pace. Even calories, if I cared to hear. But as much as I love my friend—I rarely run without her—I know she lies.

My friend's name? Nikeplus. An oval disk that sits in a divot under the footbed of my left Nike shoe (or in a little holder on the laces of my non-Nike running shoes) and a small, rectangular sensor plugged into the butt of my iPod Nano, Nikeplus tracks my runs. When I connect my Nano to the computer to charge it, all the info gets sent to nikeplus.com, making an online log of my miles and speed.

But like I said, it lies. Or rather fibs. Even after calibrating the sensor to my pace, it still overestimates how far I run and how fast. I used to get ticked off, but now I just accept the "vanity" flaw and mentally change the stats in my head. So when my pal's voice congratulates me for covering 6.86 miles in 1:00:59 with an average pace of 8:52, I know I actually covered about 6.6 miles at more than 9 minutes per mile.

I stick with my friend Nikeplus because I love perusing my slightly exaggerated runs online, and I like the integration of timekeeper and music player into one device. Plus there's an added bonus: Every so often, after my invisible gal-pal tells me my stats, Lance Armstrong purrs in my ear, "Congratulations! You've just recorded a personal best for the mile." Yeah, he lies, too, but he sounds mighty fine doing it.

think, *This feels good. Maintain this.* Four steps, and I'm back at 9:30 and fire up my jets again—and repeat the cycle for miles and miles. I'm not the only one with this affliction: I once wrote a blog about it, and a runner wrote back, "The other day, I strapped my Garmin to my dog's collar so that I wouldn't look at it. But even way down on her neck, I stopped to take a peek about three times a mile. Then I'd think, 'You slowed down, now you have to make up for your little stop! Run faster!' I'm addicted."

Needless to say, the Garmin has the potential to suck the life out of a run.

The good news is, you can program it to smooth out the hills and average your pace (however, I'd have to open the manual or at least talk to a more tech-savvy running pal to figure out how). And the feedback really is helpful, both as a distraction and as a tool for getting fitter and faster. I wear it now on two out of three runs, chilling out with my trusty Timex on the other one. Like wine and reality television, it's best in moderation.

GLOVES

As much as people spout off about 90 percent of your heat being lost through your head, gloves are the key to warmth on a run. (My very unscientific proof? All the elite marathoners who dress in a skimpy singlet, split shorts, and five-fingered heat holders for fall races.) Find a pair that's fairly thin and made of synthetic material. Liners you wear under ski mittens can work well in a pinch, but they lack the oft-needed snot swiper, a terry cloth patch on the thumb and forefingers, found on most true running gloves. I don't know about you, but if I could run as fast as my nose does on chilly days, I'd be winning my age group.

SUNGLASSES

Being blinded by the light when the rest of your body already feels *en fuego* feels almost insulting: I have to run up this hellish hill and now I can't even see it? Thanks, universe. Stash a pair of shades on the top of your head or over the brim of your cap so you can have the last laugh. Once they're on your face, if they fog up when you take a pit stop, pull them down to the tip of your nose for 30 seconds or so to clear them, then push them back.

Find a pair that stays put behind your ears and against your nose so you're not constantly doing the daft professor thing and pushing them back up. Things to look for: gripping rubber on the nose-bridge and temples, full coverage around your eyes, UVA and UVB protection, shatterproof lenses, and—perhaps the hardest assignment—a style that doesn't scream *Terminator*.

HAT

No matter the season, my running lid never wavers: an athletic baseball hat. I run too hot to sport a knit hat ever. I'm as picky about my hat as I am about my choice of diet soda (Caffeine Free Diet Coke, in case you're wondering). It needs a generous brim so I'm shaded from the rain (and occasional sun, when it peeks through); an adjustable strap, as I have a mop of thick hair and a melon head; enough ventilation to keep my head cool but not so much that rain soaks me; and a band that pulls sweat off my brow, as I'm a sweaty-Betty. And the depth of the ideal hat is crucial. For me, most running hats, especially ones designed for women, are too shallow. They sit on my mound of unbrushed hair like a beanie, ready to blow off in the slightest whiff of wind. But swing too far to the deep end, and the hat turns me into a trucker wannabe, which I don't wanna be.

It's all a tall order, I know. No wonder I have a rack full of hats but always reach for the same one or two. They are salt-stained, tattered companions that have covered almost as many miles as I have.

—Sarah

Ditto what she said, except I rotate between a baseball hat (summer), a thin fleece knit hat (winter), and a bandana–sunglass combo (fall and spring). Running in real winter temps—not the faux winters of the Pacific Northwest—demands ear protection. Plus, I love coming home from a run when it was freezing outside and seeing the one-of-a-kind ice sculpture, created with sweat, over my forehead.

—Dimity

EXTRA TRACTION

If you're running over any surface that is remotely slick during the winter, invest in a pair of Yaktrax or Kahtoola Microspikes, the equivalent of tire chains that lash on the bottom of your shoes. Doing so turns your soles from baldies to veritable studded snow tires. If you're handy with a drill, you can insert screws into your shoes for extra traction (Google "screw shoe"), but whatever you do, take it from my formerly broken wrist, shattered when I slipped on ice: Beef up your soles.

SUNSCREEN

I'm ridiculously obsessed about my children's skin—I've thought about lathering Amelia's armpits before school, in case she spends the entire recess on the monkey bars—but am haphazard, at best, about my own epidermis. I kid myself that the early morning sun doesn't feel so hot or I'm only going out for 30 minutes, so sunscreen won't make a difference. It does, as Olympic marathon bronze medalist Deena Kastor can attest. A skin cancer survivor, Kastor doesn't go for a run without sunscreen and a hat, and she usually doesn't leave her doctor's office without some menacing mole being biopsied or removed. Even if you don't have her fair skin, think big picture: It's not just your face getting hit by the sun. Your back needs it if you're wearing a tank, your knees need it, the tops of your ears need it.

PRACTICAL *Motherly* ADVICE
NEED IT OR LEAVE IT? AN ACCESSORY CHEAT SHEET

	30 MINUTES	60 MINUTES	90 MINUTES	2+ HOURS	CAVEAT
CELL PHONE				✓	Take it on any run if it makes you feel more at ease. And always take it on trail runs.
HYDRATION		✓	✓	✓	An hour run depends on weather; details in Chapter 15.
ID	✓	✓	✓	✓	Buy a personalized one, worn around your wrist, at roadid.com, and stash it in your shoes after a run so you remember to put it on.
CALORIES			✓	✓	Chapter 15 is your guide.
SUNSCREEN	✓	✓	✓	✓	You're only off the hook if a) it's December, it's cloudy, and you live north of the Mason–Dixon line; b) it's raining; or c) it's dark out.
CASH		✓	✓	✓	A few dollars is enough for a phone call, refreshments, or the start of a taxi ride home.
BODYGLIDE OR VASELINE			✓	✓	Coat your inner thighs, pits, underneath your sports bra straps, anything with the potential for chafing.

Sport sunscreens seem to work best, but apply wisely, especially around your eyes; a combo of sunscreen and sweat often creates burning eyeballs, which feels about as pleasant as it sounds. A hat with a wide, sweat-soaking brim seems to stop most of the flow and has the added benefit of extra sun protection. Two random pieces of advice I've learned the hard way: Use the bottom half of your shirt, not your sunscreen-coated arms or hands, to wipe sweat off your face, and don't apply Neutrogena Healthy Skin Eye Cream before bed the night before a run. It only took me, like, five runs in tears to finally make the connection.

HYDRATION

Water transport is one of the trickiest issues when it comes to longer training runs. The farther you go, the more you need to drink; the more you need to drink, the heavier your load becomes. Short of turning into a camel, there's no easy way to carry it. But there are three options:

• In your hands, either with or without a carrying strap around the bottle
  PROS: Easy access. No chafing or extra weight from carriers.
  CONS: Water heats up quickly in your hands. Lopsided weight in one hand can throw your stride a little off kilter and cause forearm strain. No extra pockets for keys or phone on the bottle itself, although some carriers have them.

• Around your waist
  PROS: Extra pockets. Easy to center the weight of the water. Can carry one or two 16- or 24-ounce bottles or four or five 8-ounce mini-bottles.
  CONS: Bottle easy to pull out but can be tricky to replace behind you while running. Some belts are hard to adjust correctly, so there's potential for jostling with every step. A slice of nerdiness.

• On your back
  PROS: Pack is spacious enough to stash a change of clothes. Hauls enough water for a marathon training run and recovery afterward. Convenient tube for drinking. Plenty of straps to keep it tight and centered.
  CONS: Overkill, especially if you're running in a race or on a route with plenty of water stops. Water can heat up quickly when it's against your back. Extra weight of water and pack.

I carry my drink in my hands with a tight neoprene holder over the bottle, while Sarah, who ran the Nike Marathon with a Camelbak, now prefers a FuelBelt, which holds 40 ounces of water in minibottles. She doesn't like the idea of running out of water, but I'd rather go thirsty than haul one extra ounce.

.2 COMMERCIAL PROPOSAL
CLIENT: WIN DETERGENT
WRITER: SARAH BOWEN SHEA

Win Green Detergent: *It Makes Good Scents*

(30 seconds)

VIDEO: *Toned, tanned couple embracing after a road race. They are glowing with love—and perspiration. The all-American-looking dad takes his hand off the handle of a jogging stroller to wipe sweat off his glistening brow. Asleep in the stroller is a cherubic 15-month-old baby clutching a well-loved, crumpled, blue, green, and white striped blanket.*

VOICEOVER: Nothing feels quite as good as pushing yourself. To be the best you can be. And to share the experience with your whole family.

VIDEO: *Wife of couple, dressed in white capris, striped tee, and wedge flip-flops, taking race outfits out of hamper. Her strong reaction—grimacing and waving hand in front of nose—shows she's repelled by the odor of the workout wear. Then she pulls the striped fleece blankie from the bottom of the hamper, and she doubles over from the stench.*

VOICEOVER: Yet it's no fun to share that God-awful stink that overcomes you when you take sweaty clothes out of the hamper or gym bag after they've been festering for days. Admit it: Your stuff ferments for days. By then, the bacteria have been feasting on the sweat, leaving behind their stinky mess. The only thing that smells worse is the wretched odor of your child's sucked-on, slept-on, sneezed-on lovey, which he has been unwilling to have washed for more than 6 months.

VIDEO: *Wife looking perplexed as she stands in front of new, gleaming, low-energy washer–dryer. She picks up a small, white bottle of laundry detergent. As she reads the label, a smile starts to creep across her face.*

VOICEOVER: The solution for both? Win Green, a dye- and fragrance-free laundry detergent that kills even the stinkiest odors in your workout clothes and the beloved blankie or stuffed monkey you bribe your kid to part with for one wash cycle. Powerful oxygenated technology goes deep into the fibers to remove sweat, spit, puke, poop, baby food, and all the other cling-ons making you gag.

VIDEO: *Close-up of bottle of laundry detergent.*

VOICEOVER: Win Green: It makes good scents for your whole family. Go to sportdetergent.com to smell for yourself.

07

MUSIC: GIMME A BEAT

By Sarah

In the 1990s, I went through a purist phase when I believed real runners don't listen to music. I copped this elitist attitude after hearing that Dana, the wife of my good friend Allen, ran sans music. Dana, now the mother of three preteen boys, is one of the people who inspired me to run marathons. I was in awe of her for training for 26.2 while living on Bermuda. (Talk about monotonous: I imagine there are, at most, two long-run routes on the island.) To me, she was a goddess on par with Atalanta; she ran the Boston Marathon, then immediately hopped on a plane, clad in her sweaty tee, shorts, and a Mylar blanket, to get to a meeting in NYC. She was everything I wanted to be. So when I heard she scoffed at music, I ditched my Walkman.

Maybe because music was so clunky back then, I enjoyed the freedom and liberation I felt as I clipped along with only the wind in my ears. It seemed safer to run without distractions, able to hear traffic and people around me. I felt I was more serious about my training because I focused on the motion and exertion of running instead of being distracted by a 10,000 Maniacs tape. I fancied I was a more contemplative person because I could keep my mind occupied for an hour (or more) every day.

Yet, in reality, I was bored. Looking back, I have no clue how I made it through training for three marathons without tunes. Once I tried an iPod Nano in the summer of 2006, there was no turning back for me. You mean I could hear the Weather Girls' "It's Raining Men" without having to sing it, off-key, myself? On my first run with tunes, I meant to go only 4 miles, but time flew. I was 3 miles from home before I realized I should turn back. And I haven't turned back, in the metaphoric sense, since. I now always listen to music when I run, even—insert collective gasp here—on the trail.

Yet that doesn't mean I wasn't stuck in a previous decade. Midway through my 50-minute run yesterday, Meat Loaf's classic "Paradise by the Dashboard Light" shuffled onto my iPod, and immediately my pace—and my pulse—quickened. Whenever I hear that song, I am immediately catapulted back to sixth grade, when my good friend Amy and I thought it was *sooooo* scandalous.

And now our bodies are oh so close and tight
It never felt so good, it never felt so right

Meat Loaf is just one of the mortifying music choices I'm owning up to. My iPod is full of music from the late 1970s through the late 1980s. Culture Club, Hoodoo Gurus, Duran Duran, Alphaville, and the Human League. Heck, it would be loaded with even more New Wave music except that all my high school music is on vinyl.

I'm not hopelessly mired in the past. I am hip to other areas of pop culture; my favorite magazine is *Entertainment Weekly* (yes, I love it even more than *Runner's World*). I've been addicted to *30 Rock* since Season 1, and I read *The Road* by Cormac McCarthy long before Oprah touted it. But until recently, I was out of the loop about current music: I didn't know Shakira from Shania, R. Kelly from Kelly Clarkson. I was content in my time warp, running to tunes from the years when an aging Hollywood star was president, not a vibrant African American man.

Yet a part of me wanted to jump into the twenty-first century, music-wise. What pushed me over the edge was a Facebook comment made by my buddy Shannon, another twin-mommy marathoner. It was in her "25 Random Things" lists everyone was doing in early 2009. Along with "I'm not very opinionated" and "Taking a nap is like heaven for me," she wrote, "I can't keep up to date with modern music. There's too much of it, and I can't bother to spend the time to find what I like, so I tend to stick with what I know." I often felt the same way, yet reading it on Facebook made it seem as frumpy as a pair of high-waisted "mommy jeans." That was it: I vowed to leave Simon LeBon in the dust.

But where to start? I began the way all women make important decisions: I asked my friends. Dear Dimity turned me on to the Dixie Chicks (for which I'm eternally grateful!) and some current Bruce Springsteen. Marissa burned me a Girl Talk CD. Naomi turned me on to 2pac. Several buddies suggested electronica, but that music made me want to run away, not faster.

Given that I lead the semi-hermetic life of a writer, I quickly realized I needed to extend my music search further. So I started using my Facebook status. I bared my out-of-date soul and typed, "Sarah Bowen Shea just discovered the joy of running to Rihanna, and she's looking for similar bounce-along songs." Mom-of-one Katie answered my plea, recommending Brandy's "Right Here (Departed)," and I'm forever indebted to her. That single suggestion—and a high-tech innovation or two—opened up a whole new world for me.

TAKE IT *From* A MOTHER
WHAT MUSIC FIRES YOU UP?

"'Smooth Criminal' by Alien Ant Farm. When I was training for an Ironman, I secretly imagined myself doing the race. I got so fired up! Now when I listen to it and remember the imaginary race, I compare it to my actual one and I'm flooded with emotion. It almost makes me cry."

—KAMI (best part of running: "the quiet, and my breathing.")

"I envision Eminem and Ludacris at the end of the trail, singing me in. Gotta look good as I bring it home for them."

—SHELLEY (knees go out at mile 8 or 9.)

"I only listen to music on the treadmill, and right now I'm totally into doing speedwork to old R&B. That sounds crazy, but I defy anyone to get on a treadmill with Lena Horne belting out, 'You've got to believe in yourself, yeah! Right from the start!' and not run like an Olympian. Her voice is its own power source."

—CHARITY (pre-run fuel: banana and coffee.)

"I like to start the run with the song 'Fat Bottomed Girls' by Queen. It just has a way of getting me motivated; I don't have the typical runner's body. It's also a fun way of reminding myself why I need to get out there and run in the first place."

—REBA (favorite flavor of GU: chocolate.)

"My current fave is 'Stronger' by Kanye West: It reminds me to strive to be 'better, faster, harder, stronger.'"

—AYNNE (started running because it smelled like spring outside.)

"I'm a very early morning runner, so I usually forgo music for safety reasons. But when I do run with tunes, it's music from the '60s and '70s—old-school rock. They make me laugh and forget the pain!"

—HOLLY (mantra: If it were easy, everybody would do it.)

"The song 'Thanks and Praise' by G. Love. It makes me grateful for my strong, healthy body."

—DANA (doesn't race because "I'm competitive in other areas of my life.")

"'Loud' by Big and Rich gets me fired up! I played it over and over during the later miles of my first marathon. I just focused on the loud beat and on getting the job done."

—AMANDA (surprise Christmas present to her family: a trip to Disney World so she could run the marathon.)

"It's hard to find a reggae song to run to, but 'Now That We Found Love' by Third World works. It brings me back to college days, when I could click off the miles without worrying about sore knees or a nagging back."

—TRACY (works with much more focus after a run.)

In a moment of inspiration, I created a "Brandy" station on Pandora (Pandora.com), which serves up songs based on the melody, rhythm, lyrics, and such of the favorite songs or bands you plug in. No idea who thought of that, but I love him or her. From that one song, 3 minutes, 38 seconds long, by a teen sensation, I was introduced to the Black Eyed Peas, Beyoncé, and Britney Spears. (Like I said, I was woefully stuck in the last millennium.) This wasn't music I'd listen to if I ever had the chance to just sit around and enjoy music—I think I had that luxury back in the day, if I remember correctly—but, for me, Brit and Co. create the perfect running tuneage. Upbeat, catchy, fast-paced, inane.

Another techy way I was exposed to more new music is through coached runs from Nike Sport Music (search for Nike Sport Music in iTunes Store). The 30- to 45-minute workouts feature star athletes guiding you through a run while power songs rev you up. Nothing quite like Serena Williams telling me, "Part of training is making your mind just as tough as your body," to make me go faster and farther. Doing Serena's Spontaneous Speed workout, I discovered one of my all-time favorite tempo songs: "Just Fine" by Mary J. Blige. I can't help but pick it up when she belts in my ear.

The timing for my musical epiphany was perfect; it happened when I was training for my most recent marathon. My very tired, Reagan-era favorites were making my feet feel heavy and my legs leaden. But as soon as Flo Rida's "Right Round" or Ciara's "Love Sex Magic" started playing, my feet flew. Realizing I could capitalize on that effect, I started packing my marathon playlist full of my new favorites—then didn't listen to the mix until marathon day. I wanted the songs to be fresh and

Run LIKE THIS MOTHER
LOSE THE TUNES

By Dimity

At the risk of sounding like a tsk-tsking grandmother, I say "No music at races." I'm far from an old-school runner; I embrace all technology, including my well-worn Nano, and the distraction and motivation it gives me. And I honestly don't care if the Pump-It-Up playlist you have blaring in your ears spurs you to finish 2 minutes faster than me.

What I do care about, though, is that music creates a bubble around you. It inhibits the camaraderie that begins with the thunder of thousands of footfalls at the starting line and is carried through the length of the race with occasional chatter. Don't worry: I'm not the annoying person who never shuts up, but I do like to use my mouth for more than just breathing during a race. Depending on the circumstances, my talk might range from muttering, "Nice job," as somebody passes me to having a lengthy discussion of the last half-marathon somebody recently ran. The conversation is never deep, but it cements a connection between runners, a breed of typically solitary people who can talk about black toenails without getting grossed out, hill repeats without asking why you do them, and 5 A.M. alarms without questioning your sanity.

Sometimes, but not often, I may not even say a word. But having an option to communicate is part of what makes a race a party of sorts for our self-selected community. Even if the volume on your music is low, the message your headphones send is clear: I'm running my own race.

invigorating during the race. It worked like a charm: I knocked more than 8 minutes off my previous personal best. (OK, a little speedwork helped the cause as well.)

Since getting tuned in and turned on, I'm now open to other styles of music. I've branched out from hip-hop and R&B into new realms. It's like exploring running routes during a trip to see relatives, an invigorating break from the mundane. I've added some Johnny Cash into the mix, along with songs from headbanger hair bands such as Poison, AC/DC, and Whitesnake. When "Here I Go Again" cycles onto my iPod while I'm checking e-mail, I have to restrain myself from heading out for a run, or at least pumping my fist rhythmically in the air while bobbing my head.

With that admission, I realize I may be headed for another, scarier '80s rut. For now, though, I'm looking forward to the day when my kids can recommend music to me. I recently reconnected with my "Paradise by the Dashboard Light" pal Amy, who is now a triathlete with boy–girl twins and an older daughter, just like me. (Scary how that works out sometimes.) The other day we got into a round of Facebook messages in which she told me, "If I didn't have a teenager and two tweens and I didn't manage the family iTunes folder, I'd have no idea who any of the 'cool' bands are." She went on to suggest I check out songs by the Ting Tings, Freezepop, and Pitbull. They are a little too out-there for me right now, but give me time. At this point, I think I'm stuck at about 2007.

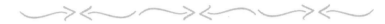

.2 I HEART ZAC EFRON
By Sarah

I'm saying it loud, and I'm saying it proud: I sing along to *High School Musical* songs when I run. "Just Wanna Be with You" from *High School Musical 3* was in the mix that propelled me to a half-marathon personal best. "Everyday," the finale in *HSM2*, lifts my spirits—and gets my feet moving—when I'm dragging. And "We're All In This Together" from the original totally sums up how I feel at a crowded starting line.

If HSM makes your skin crawl, you don't have to sprint to the other end of the age-range for Raffi. (I've sung "Baby Beluga" enough in my life to never hear it again, thanks.) There's a flock of groovy children's artists out there—Dan Zanes and Justin Roberts are two of Dimity's favorites—and plenty of former adult artists who had kids and couldn't stay away from singing about dinosaurs and bath time. (Cake, They Might Be Giants, and Barenaked Ladies, to name a few, have all taken the leap.) And why not? Kids' songs typically have an upbeat tempo. Their lyrics, often written for the enjoyment of the adults, can be hilarious. ("It's not naptime now," croons Roberts, "So don't even start with those carpet squares.") And they usually carry an uplifting message, which can prove useful during rough patches.

Another kid song I love to run to is from the TV show Yo Gabba Gabba: "Lovely, Love My Family" by The Roots. Its punchy rhythm gets me quick-stepping no matter how early or dark it is, and the lyrics hit home. "The sun shines bright and I feel peace like nowhere else/I know I'm in good health and life keeps going, I keep moving, I'm alright."

And every time John Lennon's lilting version of "Blackbird," not exactly a kid's song but close enough, swings into rotation, it nearly stops me in my tracks. The lullaby reminds me of nursing my three babies, a memory that makes me feel more powerful than Eminem ever could.

08

RUNNING PARTNERS: **FRIENDS, INDEED**

By Dimity

I first spotted Katherine at toddler time at the library. Ben, suspended off my shoulders in a Bjorn, was six-ish weeks and Amelia, at 3 years old, was the perfect age to be enchanted by the abrasive voices the librarian was giving to her hand puppets. We had just moved to Colorado Springs, where I knew exactly one adult, Grant, and longed for a girlfriend more intensely than I craved four continuous hours of sleep. Trying to divert my attention from the squawking, I noticed Katherine's red pixie hair—a rarity in the Springs, where traditional values and hairstyles reign—and her outfit, which was something along the lines of a fitted tee, capris, and ballet flats. Sitting across the room, with my cropped hair, decidedly not fitted tee (I was happy just to be out of my maternity wear), capris, and flip-flops, I mentally connected us. Whether or not she knew it, she was *going* to be my friend.

At the end of the torturous "If You're Happy and You Know it," the puppets were finally laid to rest. I sidled up to her and her two girls and used the hackneyed mom pick-up line, "How old are your cute girls?" Turns out, *They were just a few months younger than Amelia!* and *Wow! They're twins even though one is blonde and one is a redhead!* and *Does that happen often?* and *Do twins run in your family?* and *My name is Dimity!* and *Yes, I just moved here!* and *Wow! We live close to each other!* and *Yes! I would love to get your number and hang out!* Ben, sick of being a Roo on my chest, started fussing about 5 minutes into my verbal diarrhea, so we packed up. The thought of stalking her—or at least following her home to see how truly close we lived—crossed my mind.

Fast forward about 6 months. I started contemplating a marathon, for the main reason an underslept, overambitious mother typically does: She wants a few free moments in her day when she's not doing something—folding the laundry, writing a memo, heating up a bottle—for somebody else. I ran the idea past another newish friend, a seasoned runner who hadn't conquered 26.2 or childbirth yet, but she replied with a vague, "Sounds good," which really meant, "Not interested." Knowing I wasn't mentally prepared to deal with the demanding training schedule solo—I wanted alone time, but not *that* much alone time—I put the idea on hold. Then Sarah and I lucked into our marathon assignment, and there was no turning back. So I asked Katherine, who had been a runner as a teenager, to join me. She had every reason to say no: two kids, a part-time job as an attorney, plenty of friends and social dates, a husband who, though generally supportive of her, wasn't thrilled with the idea of solo Sunday mornings while she was on a long run.

But she said yes. *Yes!* This person, whom I liked more every time I saw her, wanted to commit to run a very long, long way with me and see me on a nearly daily basis? I couldn't believe it. Scared she'd back out once she saw the 5-month training schedule and grasped its exhausting implications, I bought her an iPod Shuffle for her birthday and loaded it with everything from Moby to Madonna. I figured she could use it on those few occasions we wouldn't be able to run together or after our conversation trickled out 90 minutes into a long run.

For 2 months, I'd pick her up, either on foot or in my minivan, and we'd start our days together. The morning air was cool, the streets were empty, and our chatter was endless. You name it, we covered it: the merits of Montessori; our favorite parts of the book *Eat, Pray, Love* (the pray part, if you care); tough family relationships (often cliffhanger convos that continued from one run to the next); ridiculous fights with (temporarily) unreasonable husbands; the McDonald's chocolate shake I could almost taste and was definitely buying after I showered; life decisions we'd change if we had the chance. She hardly turned on her Shuffle. And I, an independent person who likes a wide circle of space around her, never got sick of her. In fact, in a matter of months, she became one of the closest girlfriends I've ever had. Running is conducive to frank, sometimes soul-baring conversations in the same way road trips are: When you keep your eyes on the road, you can speak from your heart.

Every mile was easier—not easy, but easier—because she, a lithe, natural athlete who happened to be the granddaughter of an Olympic medalist in the 800 meters, reigned in her lean legs and stayed with me. I'd tell her I was cooked, and she somehow convinced me to keep going. I'd tell her I *really* needed a walk break, and she agreed to walk with me. About 30 seconds into it, I'd feel guilty for slowing her and pick it up again. She'd mention the snow on the top of Pike's Peak in late June, and I'd remember to keep my eyes up, not down. I'd tell her to just go ahead, that this pace was as fast as I could handle. Sometimes she obeyed me, and sometimes she didn't. Either way, I knew she was there with me for the entire journey.

Our differences in natural talent were most apparent when I chased her up impossible hills. At the top of one, she nicely asked me, "Are you OK?" My response: "No." *Wheeze.* "But." *Wheeze.* "Yes."

TAKE IT *From* A MOTHER
DO YOU RUN WITH A PARTNER, GROUP, OR DOG?

"I run with my local group twice a week. It especially helps to motivate me during the winter, because I feel like I have a commitment I need to honor. The runners I've met through it have inspired me and helped me more than they realize."

—AYNNE (while training for a marathon, she asked her non-running pals to find their own personal marathon, "something that challenged them and benefited them or others.")

"I always prefer to run with a partner. Conversation passes the time and deepens the relationship. They can also pull you through rough patches."

—TAMARA ("If I could run anywhere in the world, it would be alongside my twin sister.")

"All of the above. I like having a partner because it keeps you accountable, more than a group does. I also like groups, though, because if someone doesn't show up, you're not alone. Going with a dog kills two birds with one stone: You both get a great workout, and no need for the dog park later."

—SHERYL (current goal: to do one pull-up before she gets pregnant again.)

"None of the above. I sometimes join a group for a weekend long run, but it's hard to fit that in and still fit in family time, so I do a lot of solo training."

—RAQUEL (husband ran a marathon with her the day after he ran a half-marathon. "His recovery pace is a tad faster than my tempo pace.")

"My dog, a 90-pound boxer I got so he could run with me."

—SARA (her co-workers call her extreme. "Which is funny, because most runners would think I am normal.")

"A group, for many reasons: It motivates me, gives me a chance to be social and makes me feel safe running in the morning."

—VALERIE (worst parts of a run: getting out the door and last half mile.)

"I run with a club. It's become such a special group of women. We obviously have common goals and interests, and nobody is obnoxiously competitive. Well, there was one, but we ousted her."

—MELISSA (best core move: hanging leg lifts. "They make you use your core because you have to focus on not swinging your legs while you lift them.")

> *"I recently started a moms' running club, and we do group runs. Sometimes it hinders me to run with somebody, because I feel like I'm holding them back or because chit-chat is not my favorite thing when running. I do like somebody who helps me keep on a pace goal, though."*
>
> —NAOMI (her club's babysitting strategy: one member watches the kids while the other moms run near that member's house.)

Wheeze. She thought that was hilarious: "That's our marathon slogan! 'No but yes'! We'll print it on T-shirts!," she yelled without even taking a breath. My lungs and legs hated how easy hers made running look, but I was so grateful for our deepening friendship and her spirit, I would've tried to slash another 30 seconds off my average pace just to hang with her.

Long story short: I got a stress fracture in my heel. We trained alone for 2 months: her on the road, me on the bike, both of us with tunes blaring. She checked in on me nearly daily, letting me bitch about pedaling nowhere. Then she floated across the finish line in under 4 hours, and my pride for her was nearly maternal. We spent the post-marathon day shopping in San Francisco, reliving our races as we browsed and laughed.

And then, as typical underslept, overtrained mothers are prone to do after finishing a marathon, we stopped running. The post-race blues set in hard for me: no daily reason to run, no daily Katherine. We had coffee and playdates, but kids, cell phones, and other tasks of life constantly interrupted. Nothing felt as fulfilling and true as our daily shared sweat sessions at the crack of dawn. (A shared bottle of wine on a Friday night came the closest, but a hangover and an endorphin rush aren't really comparable.)

I wish this story had a movie-worthy ending, that we planned another marathon together or at least kept up regular runs. But she had a whiny hip, I was more interested in triathlons than straight running, and our exercise paths diverged. So our warp-speed friendship dialed back to the pace of a regular one: phone calls every third day or so, weeks going by without seeing each other, not being fully versed in the minutiae of each other's daily life. The few times we did get back out there together, though, our footfalls and chatter fell in sync easily. Those runs were bittersweet, like having one bite of to-die-for carrot cake. Yes, I appreciate that bite, but dang it if I don't want a whole hunk of it.

In my heart, though, I know our friendship will never be truly regular. I mean, how could it be when we've traveled hundreds of miles together at speeds that invited fluid conversation and always ended in appreciation?

PRACTICAL *Motherly* ADVICE
SIZING UP POTENTIAL TRAINING BUDDIES

I wasn't imagining the effect of Katherine's presence in believing I could lower my average pace; science backs me up. Researchers at the University of Virginia stood at the bottom of a hill, which had a 26-degree grade. They loaded up thirty-four students with a backpack that held about 20 percent of their body weight, then asked them to estimate the steepness of the hill; some of the students had friends standing next to them, others were alone. Those with a pal guessed the hill to be less steep than those who were solo. What's more, of the pairs of friends, the length of friendship also correlated with the lowest estimates of the hills.

Less perceived effort, more distraction, a faster pace than you're used to: What's not to love about making running as collaborative as possible? I've sampled all varieties of partners, and here are some pros and cons to each:

POTENTIAL TEAMMATE: A COACH
Top Three

1 Serious accountability, both personal and financial (if I'm paying for these workouts, I'm doing them!).

2 Deep knowledge of training coach presumably has and can apply to your schedule when things go awry.

3 Instant cachet at races and with other running friends: "My coach told me to. . . ."

Bottom Three

1 Cash. Hard to justify a coach for yourself on monthly household family budget.

2 Serious accountability. (Pick your coach wisely. I suggest another athletic mother so she'll be relatively sympathetic to your why-I-couldn't-do-it-today excuses.)

3 Limits your opportunities to just go for an easy run with a random friend. Workouts tend to be preordained and purposeful.

POTENTIAL TEAMMATE: A FRIEND
Top Three
1 Vicariously living through her makes for great distraction from the run.

2 She comes cheap. (Oh, I meant it costs nothing to run with her.)

3 A bond created between you that, with miles traveled, can rival Super Glue.

Bottom Three
1 Disparate personalities—a social butterfly and a coyote who have nothing in common, for instance—can make a run more painful than it needs to be.

2 Differing ideas of what punctual means. If the plan is to meet in my driveway at 6:15 A.M., 6:18 is acceptable. 6:30 is not.

3 Speeds need to be similar; nothing says "I hate running" more than running with a pal who is chatting easily while you can't even squeeze out a "yes."

POTENTIAL TEAMMATE: A GROUP
Top Three
1 Built-in momentum. With the exception of super-small groups, it's pretty much a given somebody will show up for a scheduled run.

2 A mixture of people and paces means you're likely to find a match.

3 Instant cheering squad at local races, especially if your group membership includes a team jersey.

Bottom Three
1 The first few encounters with the group are like those awkward walks into a cocktail party alone: You scan the crowd, wonder on whom to sic yourself.

2 Cash. Some training groups require fundraising, usually for disease prevention or research. These causes are definitely worthy, but I really don't have time to raise $2,500 while

continued on page 66

I'm also "helping" my daughter sell wrapping paper for her school (read: forcing all my relatives to buy at least three rolls) and making crafts for my son's preschool to sell at an auction.

3   Lack of accountability. Some groups can get so big, nobody notices if you oversleep.

POTENTIAL TEAMMATE: A DOG

Top Three

1   Always available and willing to run.

2   Never whines about a workout.

3   Assuming your dog isn't the size or shape of a chicken nugget, she helps ward off potential predators.

Bottom Three

1   Poop and how to dispose of it without getting grossed out. (My best trick: Run an out-and-back with a dog. When she unloads, bag it, leave it on the way out, and pick it up on the way back.)

2   Envy. Four legs and a sleek torso make them much more capable, natural runners than humans.

3   Leash = potential for tangling and tripping.

.2 JAM FOR THE LADIES

There's something just groovy and empowering about listening to an all-chick playlist on a run. Or at least we think so. Here are our faves:

"Jam for the Ladies" by Moby (a man kicks it off, but Moby is a sensitive, new-age man.)

"Long Time Gone" by the Dixie Chicks

"Freeway" by Aimee Mann

"Suddenly I See" by KT Tunstall

"My Moon My Man" by Feist

"Stronger" by Britney Spears

"Power to the Meek" by the Eurythmics

"Heartache for Everyone" by the Indigo Girls

"Right in Time" by Lucinda Williams

"Light Enough to Travel" by the Be Good Tanyas

"4 Minutes" by Madonna (featuring Justin Timberlake and Timbaland)

"Disturbia" by Rihanna

"Whenever, Wherever" by Shakira

"Head over Heels" by the Go-Go's

"My Life Would Suck Without You" by Kelly Clarkson

"Soak Up the Sun" by Sheryl Crow

"Surrendering" by Alanis Morissette

"Change" by Tracy Chapman

"I Run for Life" by Melissa Etheridge (have to end with the anthem, of course.)

09

PROGRESSION: **EVOLUTION OF A RUNNER**

By Dimity

When I lived in New York City, I ran either around Central Park or in the gym, where I ran at lunch and immediately after work. (I knew if I even saw my couch, I'd be glued to it for the night.) Normally a rule follower, I ignored the signs posted on the walls asking users to limit their cardio time to 30 minutes. I was single, with not much to look forward to except a semi-crazy boss at work and George Clooney on *ER* at home, so a half-hour did not cut it. So I brazenly hit the 10K program choice on the treadmill, knowing full well I couldn't pull out 6.2 miles in a Kenyan-esque 30 minutes.

Conveniently, a full loop of Central Park, which I lapped in the mornings and on the weekends, was just over 6 miles long, too. I loved the neatness of both runs: a round 10K on the treadmill, a near-60 minutes in the park. I never raced and rarely sped up beyond 6.5 miles an hour. I lived in a place where my surroundings mimicked a lurching taxi ride—aggressive, loud, and potentially nausea inducing—and my five matching, weekly runs delivered an infinitesimal but crucial sense of order.

I stayed on that plateau for at least 18 months before getting up the nerve to enter the lottery for the 1997 New York City Marathon. Two years before, I stood in awe on the curb—it was the first marathon I'd ever seen—getting dizzy as wheelchair athletes, people in rhino costumes, and 30,000 other athletes flitted by. I was in such sensory overload, I hardly opened my mouth. The next year, after yelling "Looking good in the blue shirt!" or "Go Notre Dame! You can do it!" for more than 5 hours, something in me just knew I could handle it. I was young, I was injury-free. I'd run enough to know I wanted to run more. I had a couple friends who had also caught the fever, so I had a built-in support group both for training and bitching about training. Plus, the long group runs put on by the New York Road Runners Club on the weekends seemed like parties to me: Refreshments were served, people were in skin-baring outfits, single men were milling around. Of course I'd go.

Nearly 8 years had elapsed in my running life before I entered my first marathon, which may or may not be a normal time span. Unlike certain benchmarks you rely on as a mother (walking around 1 year old, uncontrollable tantrums around 3, kindergarten around 5), there is no normal when it comes to running. The only thing truly consistent among runners is that our daily runs and metaphorical journeys all start at Point A and finish at Point B.

Most running advice makes progression sound like a clear-cut set of stairs: You climb one step, hang out there, logging miles until you magically move up again, where you're guaranteed to notch another set of PRs. That may apply to the 7 percent or so of runners who have nothing but time and healthy bodies. But most of us aren't on that golden one-way escalator; we're on virtual elevators whose buttons are haphazardly mashed by a 3-year-old on his tiptoes, which means the floor on which you land is random and often not in your control. You go up and down with the seasons of the year—and those of your life. You hit your highest floor ever, feel like a rock star, then get injured and tumble back to the parking garage. You barely have the energy to look up a floor, let alone consider climbing to the next one. You hopscotch between two floors for a decade.

To prove my point—the only constant in progression is a lack thereof—here, in seven acts, is a brief recap of my unfinished journey toward Point B. At times, I've climbed with ferocity, but I've also fallen slowly, nosedived, and camped out on floor 10(K) for years. My history may not read like the next *Rocky* incarnation, but I'm betting parts of it will feel very familiar—and, as such, normal.

Act 1: In Which Dimity Learns to Run

The first week of freshman year in college, I went for a walk with my friend Courtney on the Spring Street loop, a 3-mile route. Our quads instinctively put on the brakes as we descended a San Francisco-esque hill, which Courtney's new roommate happened to be running up at the same time. Courtney made some sarcastic comment about her crazy, skinny roommate. I cracked up but was a little shocked. Call me sheltered, but until then, it never really hit me that somebody my age would run for fitness. In basketball or soccer practice, sure, but to force your 18-year-old body up a hill like that for fun? When nobody was watching you? Maybe she was crazy.

Both Courtney and I joined crew, and once our fall season was over, we started running that Spring Street loop. Wearing my first-ever pair of running shoes, a pair of Asics that I bought because—look away, Sarah—I loved their green-and-yellow grid, I tried to look the part, even though I felt like I was going to keel over.

One day, for no particular reason, I decided that hill would threaten me no longer. So I set my eyes on something about one third of the way up—probably a crushed Milwaukee's Best can—and made myself slog to it before slowing to a walk. The next time, I made it ten steps farther, and I continued to repeat the drill with ten more steps each time. Within a few weeks, I had hit the top.

I learned my first lesson about running then—break up anything seemingly impossible into small chunks—and it has carried me through nearly every mile since. On an out-and-back course, I try to think only about the "out" before worrying about the "back." A 5-mile run isn't 5 miles: It's two runs that are 22:30 long. And when all else fails, I count my steps up to 100, then start again at zero.

Senior year, in an effort to become more serious about my rowing, I started running with Carin, a non-rowing friend who used miles to minimize the effects of taters, chunks of fried potatoes that were consumed mainly at the metabolically inopportune time of 1 A.M. She led me out on a rural course with rolling hills that was probably 7 miles. My legs wobbled, but I, supposedly the athlete, somehow kept up.

Afterward, I couldn't believe she ran so far on her own. When nobody was watching?

Act 2: In Which Dimity Gets In over Her Head

My long, strong limbs supposedly provided the perfect frame for me to become an elite rower, so after graduation I spent nearly a year trying to make the Olympic squad for the 1996 Games. Within months of being in Chattanooga, the training site, I collapsed mentally because I was crumbling physically. I cried daily in the shower, the only place my teammates wouldn't see me break down.

While getting the life beat out of me—oh, I mean training three times a day—I was introduced to two helpful training concepts: going long and going fast. Our coach was a big fan of increasing aerobic capacity by building in short recovery breaks to long-ass workouts. We'd run for 20 minutes, then walk for 3, and do that 4 or 5 times. Running for 100 minutes seemed impossible to my selectively capable brain, but going for 20 was doable. I did my best to forget the "times 4 or 5" part of the workout. Amazingly, by the time the rest period was up—3 minutes sounds short but feels long enough to read a novel when you're exercising—I was ready to go again. I really liked these sessions; the goal was to keep your heart rate low, so slowness was encouraged.

We also had speed sessions at the track, where the goal was to get your heart rate higher than that of a cardiac arrest patient. We pounded through 10 × 400 or ladders (400, 800, 1,200, 1,600, and back down). I really did not like those.

PRACTICAL *Motherly* ADVICE
READY TO GET SET AND GO?

OK, you're a runner, and now you want to be a racer. Or you have enough 5K and 10K finisher's medals to melt them down and make a car chassis, but you are hankering to tackle a longer race and wonder whether you have the mettle. Jill Andre Parker, a running coach in Denver, spelled out these race-ready guidelines.

YOU'RE READY TO RUN A . . .

5K if you can run 2 miles at a time without stopping. Then, if you don't race too fast, chances are very good you can run 3.1 miles. Ideally, though, it would be better to be running about 4 days a week for about 3 miles each time.

10K if you can run about 5 miles, non-stop, feeling good. Four days of running per week is a minimum requirement, with the longest run at 5 miles, although 6 would be ideal. Your miles per week should not be less than 15 miles. If you've just completed your first 5K, give yourself about 8 more weeks of training to double the race distance.

HALF-MARATHON once you are capable of running 11 miles without stopping and you are consistently running at least 3 days a week. Training for the race, plan on running 4 or 5 days a week, with one weekly long run, one mid-distance one (5 or 6 miles), and two lower-mileage ones. You'll top out at a base mileage of about 27 to 35 miles per week. During your 2- to 3-month training, you'll build up to three long runs of at least 11 miles; the excitement of the race should pull you through the last 2 miles just fine. A novice's longest training run shouldn't exceed 14 miles.

MARATHON if you have been fairly consistently running at least 18 miles a week for 2 months or longer. It's also highly recommended to have done a half-marathon before you attempt a full one. Running 26.2 miles at one time takes some dedication; if you don't train properly, it will humble you. A first-time marathoner should allow about 20 weeks to train properly to go the distance. Use a training diary (an online one, like mapmyrun.com or runningahead.com, or a pen-and-paper version) to monitor your mileage, bumping up gradually to 40 (or more) miles per week.

TAKE IT *From* A MOTHER
WHAT DOES THE PATH OF YOUR RUNNING CAREER REMIND YOU OF?

"Like driving from New Jersey to Long Island. Roads are best traveled during off/odd hours, but even so there's a chance you'll get stuck somewhere along the way and sit for a while."

—TINA (swore she'd never do another marathon. "The last 8 miles of New York City hurt so bad. But here I am, trying to qualify for Boston in the next two years.")

"Like teaching a kid to ride a bike. Some learn to ride later than others—my running career is just 3 years old—and when you learn to ride on two wheels, you may still need a push, like a race or a running buddy, once in a while. "

—AMY (keeps kids quiet in jogging stroller with lollipops and a portable DVD player.)

"Like Madonna's career. You have to keep reinventing yourself in order to continue to get out there. Many times you are 'Borderline' in figuring out how to make time to run. Once you get out there and you finally 'Get into the Groove,' running is a bit 'Like a Prayer.'"

—TAMI ("No, I'm not a Madonna fan.")

"A light bulb in a socket. When it's first screwed in, there's some light: a little flickering. Then you tighten it all the way, and it shines brightly, clearly the focal point of a dark room. And eventually, it slowly fades. No amount of tightening can make it shine."

—DIANE (buys her shoes online. "Better value, and I don't mind having last year's colors.")

"My mom. At age 46, while working full-time and raising two kids, she ran the NYC Marathon. It took her 6 hours, and she stopped at mile 20 for a ham sandwich and a cup of coffee, but she did it. She was the epitome of 'Just do it' long before Nike told us to do it. She's showed me there's no shame in being slow or coming in last."

—MAGGIE (next goal: a half-marathon. "Someday I'll do a marathon, and I'll stop for a ham sandwich too.")

"A favorite, familiar pair of shoes. They've seen some big mud puddles (or obstacles) and some fleet-feet moments, but overall, they feel perfect every time I put them on."

—MARY (tried to restart her labor by running the hospital stairs a dozen times. "It was only three flights tall, so it wasn't much.")

"The terrain in Montana where I live: hills, mountains, rugged trails, smooth open roads."

—SHERI (hardest part of post-partum running: "Knowing what I could do before getting pregnant and starting the long climb back to get it back.")

Act 3: In Which Dimity Finds Her Happy Place

When I fled from the oarheads and moved to NYC, I promised myself I would never force any exercise down my throat again. After I came out of the shock of overtraining, I began to do what felt best: my beloved 10Ks. I didn't wear a heart rate monitor, which I basically lived in while training in Chattanooga. I didn't even use a stopwatch. I just estimated, using a traditional-faced, leather-banded watch, how long I'd run.

Two years later, I pinned on my marathon number. My basic, beginner training, a schedule I followed from the New York Road Runners Web site (nyrr.org), was all the guidance I needed. Running felt as easy to me then as it ever would be. I was focused but not intense, purposeful but not manic. It was my stability, my antidepressant, my way of tuning out the chaos of the life of an underpaid editorial flack with two roommates in a fourth-floor walkup. I still wasn't very psyched about the physical effort needed to get through a run, but I loved how I glowed afterward. Not ready to admit it out loud, I subconsciously knew my mental well-being depended on that glow.

The marathon went off without a hitch. OK, maybe one. Over miles of training, I honed this glorious image of me as I turned right on Central Park South, less than a mile from the finish. "God bless Central Park South!" I visualized myself yelling, my arms thrown up in the air. I pictured the dense crowd, in awe of my wit, erupting with applause.

Buoyed by the 25 miles already done, I sputtered out my (unfunny) line. It had rained nearly the entire race, and I was a sloppy, drowned mess. People didn't clap. They gaped. Embarrassed, I kept plodding along.

Act 4: In Which Dimity Rides the Roller Coaster

After the 'thon, I didn't want to run again for at least a month. So I didn't. And was pretty sure I'd never want to run another one, period, so I hung out on the 20-ish weekly miles floor for many years. Sometimes my mileage dipped to zero—and stayed planted there for more than a year, as I didn't really run during either pregnancy—and sometimes it inched closer to 35 when I trained for a half-marathon.

At some point in this phase, I'm not sure exactly when, I stopped swimming upstream against the idea of running. I'd finished a marathon on my own accord, so I was inexplicably drawn to some aspect of the sport. Instead of dreading most runs, I simply went on autopilot. Running became a part of who I am, how I take care of myself. I floss, I get pap smears, I choke down brussels sprouts, I run regularly.

Then Amelia came along, and the "regularly" part got tossed out with the mounds of smelly diapers. Used to being a free agent, I was freaked out by the dictatorial effect she had on my life; "I'm awake now," her eyes seemed to warn me, after her paltry 45-minute nap, "so don't you even think about doing anything else."

About a year into Amelia's life, slightly irritated at my lack of free time, I thought it the perfect time to regain my old athletic self. A training schedule and race justify time alone, right? I signed up for the Wildflower Triathlon, a half-Ironman infamous for its difficulty. I flailed through training and the cruel, cruel race. The bright side? It took only 70.3 miles of racing for me to finally accept that Dimity Version 2.0—now with new mothering skills and responsibilities!—had been installed in my body.

Then we doubled our pleasure with Ben. More diaper changing, toy wrangling, grocery shopping, parental negotiating. Much less running. I was truly depressed. I snuck out once a week or so, but my 4-mile loop was too much for my doughy body and not enough for my swirling mind. I was lonely, anxious, and angry, and had no suitable outlet to vent. (I did my best to turn Grant into a battering ram, but—dang him!—he wouldn't fight back.) I tried therapy, and the oversmiley doc suggested maybe I needed to find a mommy group. "Thanks," I thought to myself, "I can't believe I hadn't thought of that very obvious solution." I was so sick of myself, I finally gave in to what I had sworn I'd never take: meds.

Six weeks into pharmaceutically induced balance, I crept out of my hole. Figuring out how to get a run in, a task that used to seem more complicated than open-heart surgery, was no longer insurmountable. Forcing myself out of bed for 4 miles wasn't pleasant, but it was now possible. And not instantly tearing up when I slowed to a walk while running was definitely a bonus.

Act 5: In Which Dimity Stages a Comeback

The Nike marathon, which had been simmering in my head since I was pregnant with Ben, became a reality when Amelia was 4 and Ben was 1. When I look at my life—one husband, two kids, two dogs, one house, one job—through an objective lens, I see no room or reason for an athletic challenge. But that's not how I felt. Depression and deadlines be damned, I wanted something that belonged exclusively to me, that made me feel proud and vibrant. And so, another go at 26.2.

I'll admit, I had almost no memory of the training for the Big Apple when I suggested another one. And when I saw that my coach, Ivana, put a seemingly impossible 80-minute run on the schedule about 3 weeks into the program, I was ready to back out. But Katherine, my running partner, was always game, so I tried not to complain too much. Plus, the training was interesting. Long gone were my one-pace wonder days. Ivana taught me how to do tempo runs and hill repeats, both of which I found invigorating, and reintroduced me to speedwork, which was still as brutal as I remembered.

It was after five sets of 20-second strides—another new ingredient in my running kitchen—that my heel really started to ache. And, well, you know the rest of the story: stress fracture, bike, marathon, collapse. I am quite certain that was the last marathon finish line my feet will ever cross.

Act 6: In Which Dimity Challenges Herself

After fighting for 6 months to get to the point where I could get through a marathon, I thought it wouldn't be a big deal to maintain a fitness level so I could jump in a half-marathon with a month's notice or so. But that intention, like so many of my good ones—family dinners more than once a week, post-run stretches, regular date nights—inexplicably disappeared. As the fall turned to winter, my runs, hampered by an unsolvable aching glute, iliotibial band, and hip and an absent Katherine, became shorter and more painful.

Eager for some group momentum and some non-impact exercise, I joined the master's team at the local pool, signed up for power cycling classes, and silently entertained the notion of a couple sprint triathlons in the summer. That turned into four triathlons in one summer—way more ambitious than I'd ever been—and the Denver half-marathon that fall to bookend the season. For once, I gave myself a time goal, albeit a loose one: to run in under 2 hours, which I was pretty sure I'd never done before. For about 8 weeks, I trained as hard as I ever had on my own. Abby, a friend who was coaching me, had me at the track at least two mornings a week. I ran mile repeats in the 7:30-ish range. I ticked off 12-mile runs with 9 of them at a sub-8:30 pace.

On race day, for once, I had goals other than to simply get across the line happy. I was primed to slay the course. I diligently watched the mile splits on my Garmin register 8:40 or below. When an uphill mile clocked in around 9:00, I panicked and picked it up. I ran at my limit, save for walking through one water stop around mile 9, and the clock proved it. I finished in 1:52:14, faster than I ever thought I could, putting me 46th out of 484 women in the 35 to 39 age group.

Me, finish in the top 10 percent of my age group? I was thrilled. I was also beyond wiped. I knew I was headed down soon.

Act 7: In Which Dimity Slacks Off

Once again, I had no motivation to run after a big goal race. So I didn't. Then I broke my wrist, and we moved from Colorado Springs to Denver. Somewhere between packing boxes and holding garage sales, I lost what little momentum I had left. These days, I'm back on floor one, busting out 9:30 miles and logging 15 miles a week, max. For fun, I put two 10-minute tempo segments into my run the other day, and I could barely maintain an 8:40 pace during them. I wondered how I had strung together 13.1 miles faster than that less than a year ago.

But the fact that I wanted to throw those two faster miles in for "fun" means my elevator is headed up again. Whatever floor it lands on, I'll climb out and do my best to enjoy the view.

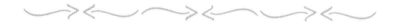

.2 TRAINING WITH THE MOUSE
By Sarah

I started getting into marathoning about the same time the mechanized AOL voice announced a gazillion times a day, "You've got mail." It was the late 1990s, I was newly divorced from my first husband, and in my free time I was racking up more miles than I ever had before. So I signed up for the San Francisco Marathon in July 1998. I'm not sure online training plans even existed then, so I improvised my training as I went along. I did a long run every weekend, but otherwise my training was haphazard.

The next year, revving up for the New York City Marathon, I decided I needed expert advice to avoid the agony I'd encountered at mile 19 in San Fran. I distinctly remember stumbling around online for a training plan—hard to believe Google didn't even exist back then—until I came across Hal Higdon's site (halhigdon.com). For NYC, I followed his Marathon Training Schedule: Novice 2 plan to the letter. I loved that it never made me run longer than 8 miles midweek, and I only had to tackle one 20-miler, 3 weeks before the race. It seemed like work, but not too much.

Oh, how my mindset has changed since then! In the new millennium, I became intent (some might say "obsessed") on breaking 4 hours, and I realized I had to put in more work than my pal Hal advised to get there. Higdon is still a safe bet for novices and even intermediates, but I think his advice is antiquated for more advanced runners. For example, he doesn't recommend embedding any marathon pace mileage into long runs. No one would mistake me for a speed demon, for sure, but I'm now aware of the value of tempo runs and track workouts. Yes, it sounds scary—and it sort of is—but running faster during segments of my long weekend runs gives me confidence I can do it during races. And it's not just a mental exercise: The work teaches my body how to sustain a faster pace well after fatigue has set in. (And we know it always does!)

So I've progressed to following Pete Pfitzinger's advice (pfitzinger.com), which has definitely ratcheted up my marathon training. "Pfitz" (say it with me: *fitz*) is all about training at marathon race pace.

For half-marathons, I'm a devotee of a 10-week plan from the August 2007 issue of *Runner's World*. I've followed the program for four half-marathons. Called Hall's Half-Marathon Training Plan (search for it on runnersworld.com), it follows the same principles as Olympic marathoner Ryan Hall did when he became the first American to run a half-marathon in less than 1 hour. I'm usually around mile 8 when Hall crosses the line, but his plan did catapult me to a 1:49:52 PR in January 2009. I'm pretty sure it's because of the Tuesday track sessions and the two longer-than-13.1-mile runs in the training program.

Training for something shorter? My good pal Dana swears by The Couch-to-5K Running Plan on Cool Running (coolrunning.com). She followed the plan herself when she returned to running postpartum, and she's recommended it to loads of novice gal-pals. She loves that it recommends runs by minutes, not miles.

Of course, there are a gazillion plans floating around out there, and many of them are very smart and helpful. But plans are like recipes. There are way too many chocolate chip cookie recipes in the world, but a few appeal best to your tastebuds. Find what works for you, then bookmark it. Or make it feel old-school: Print it out.

10

SPEED + DISTANCE: **CRANKING IT UP**

By Sarah

Ever since I was 12 years old, I've believed I might be able to go long, but never fast. I learned about muscle fibers in Mr. Manko's science class. With elaborate diagrams, he taught us slow-twitch muscle fibers are responsible for endurance, whereas fast twitch ones are, not surprisingly, the ones firing the speed boosters. I wasn't a runner yet, but from my pitiful performance in junior high basketball—I'd huff and puff to the end of the court 20 seconds after Alicia or Kim had scored yet another basket—I knew I was not built for speed.

When I started running in college, my genetic predictions seemed to play out: I often brought up the rear of the pack of rowing team novices as we jogged 3 miles to the lake, yet when we got there, I felt I still had gas in my tank while the zippier runners complained of being tapped out. After college, when I shifted from rowing to running, I accepted I had about three fast-twitch muscle fibers, compared to about three million slow-twitch ones. When I signed up for races, most were 13.1 miles. Setting my sights on going further still, I had hopes of being able to run at a decent enough clip to break 4 hours in the marathon (9:10 miles or better), but that goal proved slippery to grab hold of. I kept telling myself adrenaline would light a fire under my feet (and in my quads), but any flame I imagined always burned out around mile 19 or 20.

During the first three marathon training cycles, I vowed to do proven speed-builders such as tempo runs (warming up for a mile or two, then pushing the pace to 10 to 30 seconds slower than race pace for 3 or more miles, then cooling down for a bit) or intervals. Yet like my intentions to shave my legs more often than once a week or organize the family photos, I never quite got around to it.

After coming just 63 seconds shy of my elusive sub-4:00 goal in my third 26.2-miler, I decided it was time to get serious about speed. Knowing I needed someone to hold my Nike-shod feet to

PRACTICAL *Motherly* ADVICE
BECOME A SPEED QUEEN

Since Dimity and I aren't gazelles, we asked for advice from Lynn Jennings, who has held the women's American road-race 10K record since 1990 with a time of 31:06. Here are five style points to focus on.

- Run tall. Pretend you are a puppet and someone is pulling your strings to keep you upright. Not slanted forward, not leaning back, not collapsing onto your hips.

- Swing your arms forward to back, not across the body. Think about driving your elbows straight back behind you, then forward. The harder you drive your elbows back, the more it tells your body to lift your knees, the faster your feet move.

- Keep your wrists and hands loose, as if you are holding a baby bird or an egg. No white knuckles, please.

- Have an easy, swinging stride. Stride naturally so you are neither overstepping nor mincing along.

- Paw the ground as lightly as possible, taking light, loose footsteps. If you are slapping the ground with your feet, you're driving energy into the ground instead of propelling yourself forward.

the fire, I enlisted the help of Paula, a speedster with two teenagers and co-owner of a local running store with her marathon-winning husband. Four months before the marathon, she and I headed to a track to get a baseline to determine what constituted "fast" for me. Once I ran a timed mile, she could gauge the splits I should aim for during track workouts and tempo runs.

Doing a few warmup laps, I realized I'd run on a track only five or six times in my life, never mind four times around as fast as I could. I was petrified—and a wee bit curious to see what I was capable of. Paula told me to go at an even, hard pace. I took a final swig of water and started running.

It was surprisingly humid for a late spring day in Portland. Even before I'd hit the track, I'd been sweating from the weather—and nerves. In my second lap around the parks and rec track my forearms started to tingle. My lungs felt as if they might burst out of my gaping mouth. I concentrated on pumping my arms back and forth and lifting my knees, and the tingling sensation passed.

Run LIKE THIS MOTHER
ROUTES I DON'T TRIP OVER

When I'm in marathon-training mode, I gleefully fritter away time during my work day figuring out a route for my Sunday long run. Instead of dreading the 20 miles I need to cover, I spin an adventure in my head, daydreaming about the sights I'll see. Even though I've lived in Portland for 10 years, I'm convinced there are yet-undiscovered routes from my house. My current favorite way to find a new long run is MapMyRun.com. I'll decide on some parks I want to run by and see how far they are from my house and whether there's a scenic way to loop them together, or I hit the "Find a Run" button on the homepage and see what anonymous locals have suggested.

I rarely do the exact route they have mapped out, but through the paths of others, I've found a route to a bridge I'd never crossed on foot before and a peaceful paved trail that parallels the Columbia River and the Portland airport runways. Thank you, GetFitLiveFit and Coyote Padre, whoever you are, for your recommendations.

Before starting, I had asked Paula to write down her best guess for my mile time. "What was your prediction?" I said after I finished, in between gulps of air. "8:25," she replied. Then I asked her what my actual time was.

7:31.

I—and my three fast-twitch fibers—were overjoyed. I was ready for some speedwork.

Paula had me hit the track every Tuesday for sets of 400 meters (once around the track) interspersed with rest laps. Ten × 400 was a favorite, as was 6 × 800 meters. The intervals were challenging but short enough to be over quickly, so the pain was short lived. She wanted me to run my 400s between 1:50 and 2:00. For the first month or so, I would press the stop button on my watch at 1:58 or 1:59, but soon the numbers dropped. 1:55. 1:53. 1:51. Once, when a dad I knew from our kids' preschool, a 3:08 marathoner, was also doing laps, my ego propelled me to run 1:45. I didn't think I had it in me.

More surprising to me than my ability to improve my speed was my enjoyment of the workouts. (Caveat: *Enjoyment* is a relative term. Compared to hotel sex or a Clive Owen movie, I detested the track repeats. But I enjoyed the effort and the satisfaction of a job well done.) Instead of dreading track sessions, I found myself looking forward to them. I didn't dwell on them the night before; no reason to lose sleep obsessing how much I'd be sucking wind doing a pyramid of repeats up to a mile and back down. Instead, I'd talk myself up as I trotted over to the track and got it done. After

TAKE IT *From* A MOTHER
WHAT'S YOUR FAVORITE SPEED WORKOUT?

"1-mile warmup, 10 × 200 with 200-meter recovery, 1-mile cooldown."

—MELISSA (post-run treat: always dark chocolate.)

"Fast walking for 8 minutes to warm up, then 2 miles at 10K pace. Fast walk for half-mile followed by 1 mile at 5K pace. Fast walk for half-mile, then 2 miles at half-marathon pace. Cool down with a slow jog for 8 minutes."

—NAOMI (if I weren't running, "I'd have few options for a safe, healthy outlet.")

"Warm up for 10 minutes, or about a mile. Alternate running fast (5K race pace) for 30 seconds with going easier for 2 minutes. I continue these intervals for up to 4 miles, then cool down for 10 minutes."

—KELLI (gets through rough patches by visualizing a big rubber band attached to the person ahead of her. "I try to spring toward them.")

"Two-mile warmup, 6 × 5-minute tempo intervals (between 5K and 10K pace) with 2:30 recovery, and a couple miles for a cooldown."

SARA (dream date: running an ultramarathon with her husband in South America. "Ultras aren't about the speed but rather the enjoyment.")

"One-mile warmup, 2 miles at tempo, then 1 mile easy. Followed by 4 × 400 at 5K pace with 400-meter recovery in between. End with 1- to 2-mile cooldown. This 7- to 8-mile workout benefits both your aerobic and anaerobic systems, so it's a great one when you can only get in three runs per week."

—CHRISTINE (her husband once sacrificed his sock for emergency TP for her.)

"Speedwork on the treadmill allows me to control speed easier than the track. I do a 10-minute warmup, then 1 minute at 7:00 pace followed by 2 minutes at marathon pace. Then 2 minutes at 7:00, 2 minutes at marathon pace. I repeat this whole 1/2/2/2 series seven times total, increasing the speed with each series. End with a 10-minute cooldown—and by throwing up."

—JUNKO (strength trains after her runs. "It makes me focus, so I don't injure myself.")

TAKE IT *From* A MOTHER
WHAT'S YOUR FAVORITE DISTANCE WORKOUT?

"18 to 20 miles at an easy pace. If I can do one hard mile near the end, I feel like I can accomplish anything—though maybe not that day, exactly."

—CYNTHIA (if she could run anywhere, it would be in the Scottish Highlands. "Fog, moors, the sea, castle ruins.")

"A 12-mile trail run with some rolling hills on an autumn Saturday morning."

—ROBYN (description of her running partner: "priceless.")

"12 miles through the Rancho Penasquitos trails in San Diego with my favorite run buddy, my hubby. Remote hilly trails with a trailhead a mile from our house and views of the ocean from the hilltops. Our babysitter thinks we're crazy because we rarely call her for a Saturday date night, but instead we pay her extra to arrive early Sunday morning."

—ELI (set her half-marathon PR when her husband forgot their 4-month-old's bottle. "I ran in fear my son would be starving!")

"My current favorite is a 14.4-mile loop from my house to the Great Swamp National Wildlife Refuge, which has a 7-mile mostly dirt road mostly closed to traffic, and then back home. I often see fox, great blue herons, a flock of turkeys, and few other humans, which is remarkable for overpopulated suburban New Jersey. I can run it in just over 2 hours and still function as mom or employee (or both) afterward, without a nap."

—TISH (as she changes her clothes, her 5-year-old says, "Please don't tell me you're going to go run.")

"16 miles starting in Chico and heading out into the California countryside. I love the small-town feel, the tractors sharing the road with us, the smell of the orchards, the cute houses along the backroads."

—TINA (best race: California International Marathon, with best running buddies by her side.)

"A 12- to 15-mile, hilly trail run. Going at an easy pace but pouring it on up the hills—the flats and downhills are my recovery. Getting my heart rate up and feeling my heart pumping makes me feel powerful, like I can handle the challenges life throws my way."

—DIANE ("Ran my first marathon as a coming-of-age thing when I was 30 and I ran Boston when I turned 50. I'm done.")

a workout, I spent the day in a satisfied state, knowing I was improving on something I thought was totally outside my control. Hey, the twins might never learn to pee in the potty instead of their diapers, but at least I was making headway on the track. As the months went by, I watched my splits drop. Eventually, 400s done on 1:45 were the norm, not the adrenaline-fueled exception.

Alas, the October marathon proved too hilly to use my newly discovered speed. Disappointed yet again, I continued to train for a half-marathon 3 months later, hoping to show off my new wheels. A creature of habit, I hit the track every Tuesday into the winter, including Christmas Day. (Don't roll your eyes: I waited until the kids had opened presents.). I averaged 8:28 miles in that pancake-flat half-marathon, knocking at least 30 seconds per mile off my previous half-marathon pace. A mere 8 months after my timed mile, I became a true believer in honing speed.

For the next year, I continued doing track sessions at least three times a month, as well as the occasional tempo run. I won't lie: Sometimes I wasn't up for the hurt. But I never blew off a planned track workout. If you know me, you know that's no shocker. Me nixing a workout would be like me wearing low-cut jeans and a belly-baring halter top while doing tequila shots: not happening. Sometimes, though, my best intentions would crumple after a few repeats. It was tough to keep my motivation burning bright when I didn't have a race on the immediate horizon. A 10 × 400 workout would become 8 × 400, or I'd head home after four 800s instead of six. But my mostly consistent effort was a better investment than a Bernie Madoff hedge fund: I did the same completely flat half I had done the previous January and knocked 2 more minutes off my PR. By this point, I was clocking 400s at about 1:38 and 800s at 3:25 or so, and I still got a thrill looking at my watch after every repeat.

And I never stopped being surprised to see my faster splits because they felt the same as my slower ones. The exertion was still as great: I felt like I was pushing at about 90 to 95 percent of my max. I'm no science whiz (as my Bs in Mr. Manko's class proved), but I grasped I was notching my fitness higher by covering the same distance in less time. Maybe the thrill of getting faster pushed away boredom, or maybe it was the bouncy "Personal Best" and "5K PR" playlists I listened to exclusively on the track. No "Gold Digger" or "Wake Up Call" when I was going to be trotting along the road at 9-minute miles. Nope, those fresh songs were to get my feet moving as I went around and around.

It may sound like a joke off a Dixie Cup, but the beauty of a speed workout is that it's over—*wait for it*—quickly. When you're looking to hone your speed, there's no need to run for an hour. You can almost be done with this bang-for-your-buck workout before anyone at home notices you're gone. You don't even have to go to a track.

Head out the door and warm up for 1 to 1.5 miles. Then, on a flat stretch a block or two long, do strides. (Strides are where you amp up your speed for 20 to 30 meters, then decelerate for the same distance.) Follow this by jogging in place to get your wind back, then turn around and do the same distance strides back to where you just started. This constitutes two strides. Do six to twelve strides total, then head home.

Twenty months and at least fifty track workouts later, as I prepared for my fifth marathon, I ran another timed mile, clocking in at 6:37. With no tingling in my arms. I fluctuated between elation and disbelief. Despite having forgotten the specifics of photosynthesis, I still hear Mr. Manko's words about muscle fibers in my head. But like my complexion and my (natural) hair color, a few things have changed since seventh grade. I now believe my body can be fast.

.2   A LONG PLAYLIST FOR RUNNING LONG

When the length of a run stretches into double digits, our minds are filled with swirling sensations and flittering thoughts: a montage of ideas, memories, and emotions best summed up as, well, random. Just like this playlist. But all the tunes are mellow yet uplifting, with enough clever lyrics to stimulate your brain as your feet traipse along.

"When You're Falling" by Afro Celt Soundsystem

"In the Colors" by Ben Harper

"Catch My Disease" by Ben Lee

"Goodbye Daughters of the Revolution"
    by the Black Crowes

"The Rising" by Bruce Springsteen

"I Will Survive" by Cake

"Hard Sun (Main)" by Eddie Vedder

"Heaven Right Here (Come Over to My Yard)"
    by Jeb Loy Nichols

"Life of the Living" by Jeffrey Gaines

"All These Things That I've Done" by the Killers

"Down to Earth" by Peter Gabriel

"Skinny Love" by Bon Iver

"Snow (Hey Oh)" by the Red Hot Chili Peppers

"Such Great Heights" by the Postal Service

"I Don't Feel Like Dancin'" by the Scissor Sisters

"Viva La Vida" by Coldplay

"Read My Mind" by the Killers

"I'll Go Crazy if I Don't Go Crazy Tonight"
    by U2

"Fill Her Up" by Sting

"Between Love & Hate" by the Strokes

"Blue Ridge Laughing" by Carbon Leaf

"Grace Is Gone" by Dave Matthews Band

"When Your Mind's Made Up" by Glen Hansard
    and Markéta Irglová

"L.A. County" by Lyle Lovett

"Scare Easy" by Mudcrutch

11

HILLS: **GETTING HIGH**

By Sarah

My first year out of college I lived in one of the hilliest sections of San Francisco, which is like saying you're the tallest giant. My salary was peanuts, and I lived miles from a gym or pool, so running was my cheapo, get-it-done-before-work exercise. Almost every morning, I'd get up at 5:30 and run back and forth on the grid of city streets, climbing hills that, had they been in Lake Placid, would've been mistaken for ski jumps. (Some were so steep that cars parked perpendicular to the curb. Once, when my best friend was visiting from New York, she worried our parked car would roll over like a giant boulder while we dashed into the video store to rent *Bull Durham*.) Up and down I'd huff and puff, before the sun ever showed its face.

Looking back, I wonder what in hell I was thinking: Why did I feel the urge to climb those suckers? Why didn't I just beat my alarm clock with a baseball bat and call it a day? Then again, I now have a much more level perspective: I live on the flat side of Portland, and a 5-miler, done before the kids wake up, can easily be run with barely an incline or rise.

Traversing pancake terrain doesn't do much when you want to be a fast, strong runner. I didn't realize how helpful the ski jumps were until a friend and I jumped into the San Francisco Half Marathon and I ran it unofficially in 1:44, 5 minutes faster than my fastest in recent memory. And I do mean jumped: We decided to run it 2 days beforehand, and my longest run before that was 9 miles, max. I think it isn't age that's slowed me down (well, OK, maybe a little) but my avoidance of hills.

I suspect I'm not the only runner to take the long—and flatter—way around hills. There's a reason why there's just a vowel's difference between *hill* and *hell*. They seem so intimidating, so insurmountable, so steep, so long, so painful. I'm often not up for the self-inflicted hurt, that quad-burning, lung-exploding feeling that hits hard about halfway up and doesn't let go until the

PRACTICAL *Motherly* ADVICE
HOW TO CHARGE WITHOUT A CREDIT CARD

In my mission to tackle more hills, I've been gathering hill-climbing techniques from mountain-goat friends. Here's what I've learned:

♀ Shorten your stride and get up on your toes when you go uphill. Your body usually does this automatically, but I remind myself to stay on my forefeet as I climb. Hmmm, actually, I'd say I focus on it as I grind uphill because it stops me from obsessing about my pain going on elsewhere in my body.

♀ Drive yourself uphill with your arm swing. It adds power to your stride, which you need to propel yourself up, up, UP.

♀ Stay loose in your upper body and face. Your legs need energy, so don't waste it by hunching your shoulders, clenching your jaw, or furrowing your brow, my favorite tension spot.

♀ Concentrate. When I stop actively thinking about charging up a hill, my pace drops to a crawl.

♀ Repeat a mantra in your head or time yourself—anything to keep driving you upward. During my college crew days, I told myself if I ran fast up this one killer hill, I'd make the varsity boat. Under my breath, I'd ask myself, "How bad do you want it?" to fire me up. (Yup, *hardcore* is an adjective that gets tossed my way every so often.) And during my early morning San Francisco runs, I'd time myself up one crazy-steep hill leading back to my apartment. Knocking a few seconds off my time would make my day.

♀ Break it up. Don't charge the bottom third. Start slow, and in the middle of the hill, see if you can go a little faster.

♀ Keep your pace going up and over the hill. The hill doesn't stop at the top. Crest the sucker as quickly as you can and use the momentum to drive you downhill or across the flats.

♀ Don't put on the brakes. I'm a chicken, so the idea of leaning scares me. Instead, I tell myself to let go, to not brake with my quads on the way down. Sure, on big, gnarly descents, I rein it in, but I'm practicing letting go on longer and more gradual downhills. Give it a try.

crest is well behind me. Heck, sometimes even my neck hurts from craning to look up ahead of me! So I usually put my head down, both physically and mentally, and focus only a few yards in front of me.

Steering clear of hills was one of the things that spelled trouble for me at the Nike marathon. I'd done almost all my training on the flats because I was intent on nailing my times on tempo runs, and hitting any sort of incline messed with that goal. I was obsessed with seeing a 9:05 average pace on my Garmin at the end of every run, even though I had a nagging feeling the hills might undermine me in the race.

I rationalized it by telling myself the San Francisco Marathon—my first 26.2-miler—had only one climb in it, and I'd run that race in 4:04 with a half-assed, homegrown training plan. But in hindsight I realize I was kidding myself—and my coach, Paula. I didn't tell her about my stick-to-the-flats tactics for tempo training. So when she assured me repeatedly (because I kept asking) that I'd do fine and finally break the elusive 4-hour goal, she didn't have all the information.

The only time I was more wrong was when I thought my 2-year-old twins didn't need to wear diapers during naptime anymore.

Run LIKE THIS MOTHER
DON'T BE DECEIVED BY DOWNHILLS

By Dimity

I entered the Crested Butte 1/3 Marathon, an 8-ish mile race, a few years ago. Although the course is above 8,000 wheeze-inducing feet, it's got a major draw: The last 5 miles are downhill. *Wheeee!* I thought, *how easy is that?* Turns out, much harder than my—and most people's, I'd guess—quads can handle. The first downward mile is all smiles and jubilation: *Look, it took me less than 7:30 to run a mile!* The second mile, still flying, my knees started to complain. The third, my stomach felt like it was creating its own milkshake, whose main ingredient was puke. By the fourth, my quads toast and my head throbbing, I was ready to hang a U-turn and head back uphill. I finished, but I have never been so thrilled to see a finish line with only a slight incline. My legs were so sore, anything beyond lying prone—standing, sitting to pee, playing horsie with Ben—caused tears to come to my eyes for at least 4 days after the race.

Lesson learned: Unless you train for a downhill race, what you gain in glory (namely, a fast time), you pay for later in spades with unexpected pain.

TAKE IT *From* A MOTHER
DO YOU WALK UP HILLS?

*"Yes! Walking gives my running muscles time to recharge.
Then I can take advantage of the downhill or flat that follows
the hill, with fresher legs and controlled breathing."*

—KELLY (workout arrangement: she gets mornings, husband gets evenings.)

*"Sometimes yes, sometimes no. If the hill is really steep, I do a
fast hike up it because I can take a longer stride hiking than I can
running. But if the hill is long but not especially steep, I most often
continue to run, focusing on lifting my legs, using my quads rather
than my hamstrings. I actually get up the hill faster this way."*

—JALENE (best race memory: crossing the finish line in her first Ironman.
"Nothing will ever come close to that feeling.")

*"I used to walk, but now I only do it if absolutely necessary. What
inspires me is when I'm on the road with traffic; I imagine showing
my 'audience' how awesome I am at blowing up the hills."*

—AMY (ran her first marathon wearing a garbage bag. "It sleeted the
entire race, so I couldn't show off my new race outfit.")

*"Absolutely never. For me, those hills are like little victories over the course
of a race. I use each one as its own milestone toward the finish line and feel
some competitive adrenaline passing those who choose not to run them!
Plus, I never walk during a race, for fear I wouldn't start running again!"*

—MEGAN (really wants a buddy with a similar pace for races.)

*"I try not to. I feel so powerful pushing, pushing, pushing, then cresting, out of
breath but with a huge smile on my face. The exception is one in a crazy hill
workout our little running group does that I can't seem to conquer. I've been
going out there alone trying to tackle it by myself. It's a personal goal to get to
the top with no walk breaks before I run a half-marathon in a few months."*

—TINA (if I weren't a runner, I'd be photographing runners.)

$\mathcal{R}un$ LIKE THIS MOTHER
MY FAVORITE—OR AT LEAST MOST EFFECTIVE—
HILL WORKOUTS

If you are intent on making strength gains, hill repeats are your ticket. Don't do repeats more than once weekly—we know you're gunning to do at least three—because it turns your legs into hamburger. (But they rebound and come back as tougher hamburger, we promise.)

HILL REPEATS, THE SHORT VERSION

Find a hill that takes you at least a minute to run up and has a 5 to 10 percent grade. Not an engineering major? Me neither. A hill with an angle that's challenging, but not so steep that you're sucking wind within seconds, fits the bill. Warm up for 10 minutes, then hit the hill, thinking about charging it to maintain some speed and momentum. After topping it (whew!), resist the urge to stop, walk, or crumple to the ground. Instead, turn around and jog *slowly* down the hill—this is your oh-thank-God chance to catch your breath and to get oxygen-rich blood pumping through your hard-working muscles. Once you get to the bottom, take a deep breath, turn around, and go at it again. Start with four hill repeats, building up to ten or twelve.

HILL REPEATS, THE LONG VERSION

To turn your wheels into finely tuned machines, find a hill a quarter-mile or longer to attack once or twice during a workout. Every month or so, I head over to do an hour-long trail run that includes going up a mile-long hill twice. My pace slows by 2 or 3 minutes. But as I grind up and away, I remind myself I'm building my confidence in addition to my quads.

The marathon had 6 miles of slow, slogging hills, and I felt my selective ignorance—and wounded ego—every step of the way. One of my lowest sports moments ever happened when wait-isn't-she-slower-than-me? Dimity passed me on a steep ascent at about mile 9 of the marathon. After I gasped a few words to her, she declared, "It is what it is," and powered up the rest of the way, on stems strengthened by hilly runs at 6,000 feet elevation in Colorado Springs' Garden of the Gods park.

The hills were definitely my undoing over those 26.2 miles. Instead of finally breaking 4 hours, I ran my slowest-ever marathon (4:11). I learned my lesson. I train on hills at least once a week, and my Sunday long runs now aren't on routes as flat as I wish my abs were. Because those hills loomed large in my mind, I actually went back and re-ran the hilliest part of the Nike marathon course to prep for its half-marathon the next year.

Since then, hill repeats have become part of my monthly running plan. In a perfect world, I'd do them once a week, but until the calendar is changed to include 10-day weeks, that ain't happening. For now, I substitute in a hill workout for a visit to the track. Most mornings I stick close to home, attacking a cluster of hills about a mile from our house that climb up onto a ridge. A trifecta of hills awaits me there; the first one is slightly longer and less steep than the next two. When I do ten repeats, I typically start with three trips up the easier one, followed by three on each of the tougher hills, then I treat myself by finishing on the first, longer hill. If I'm feeling spunky, I'll toss in a few trips up and down a set of stairs sandwiched between two of the hills. This workout gives me a nice buzz, just like a handful of dark chocolate M&Ms.

When time allows—or carpooling to various camps takes me on Portland's trail-laced Westside—I attack hilly trails. They're much more challenging than my familiar trio, but I don't mind because the whole run feels like an adventure. Instead of focusing on my imploding lungs, I have to concentrate on not tripping on roots.

As for races, and especially for marathons, I now study course and elevation maps like I'm cramming for the SAT. I know exactly when each flat will turn upward like a smile. And after a quick grimace, a smile creeps across my face because I know, after I charge to the top, that there has to be a downhill somewhere ahead.

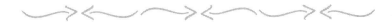

.2 FALSE FLATS
By Dimity

When you look at a false flat straight on, it doesn't even look like a hill. Then you start running on it and your calves tighten and your hamstrings complain and suddenly you're huffing more than usual. They're insidious little buggers that can kill your will to continue. They often have no real peak, and consequently they carry little sense of accomplishment. They can go on for miles and miles, or in the case of motherhood, years.

As much as I love my children, every day with the rugrats is a false flat. I start the morning, certain we're cruising on flat ground, then Ben rubs sunscreen in his eyes, Amelia can't find her other sandal, we have no bread for lunch, and Amelia chomps into Ben's back because he won't share his toy vacuum cleaner. By 8 A.M. most days, my proverbial calves are already seizing up.

Then there are the times I'm certain I'm on a false flat, and I have no idea how to end it. When Amelia was almost 5 years old and primed for the first performance of her young life—a hedgehog in a dance production of *Alice in Wonderland*—we set off to get pictures taken with her co-hedgies. We walked into the crowded building where all the performers were milling about in their costumes, and she suddenly jammed 95 percent of her hand, fingers and all, in her mouth.

I'd seen that eat-my-fist move plenty of times before and know what it's code for: I'm scared and shy and won't cooperate. So I took her to a quiet corner, dressed her in her brown finery, and tried to coax her out of her hole. She wouldn't come. I had a couple of her friends convince her to join the group. The hand stayed in her mouth. I asked her dance teacher to talk to her. Still, nothing. I offered ice cream after the picture, and when that didn't work, I picked her up and carried her into the studio, screaming. Walking by parents whose kids were predictably cooperating, I felt judged, stupid, and unsure of my mothering skills. Embarrassed by her behavior and, more importantly, by mine—really? I'm forcing my 4-year-old to take a picture, on an ugly studio backdrop, that I probably won't even buy?—I finally relented and we went home, picture-less. Mentally, I generously gave her 50/50 odds she'd make it onto the stage come performance night.

I thought Amelia had made serious headway into her shyness, that it had leveled out. She went back with the dental assistant to get her teeth cleaned alone; I waited in the office. She no longer sat out swimming lessons. She even occasionally tossed a "hi" to a stranger as she passed her on the bike path. And this situation was pretty familiar—it was her normal dance studio, teacher, and class—and we'd been talking hedgehogs for months.

But that day, she reminded me, when she encounters unfamiliar territory, the road ahead continues to be anything but flat. And the hardest thing for me, as a mother, is that I can't climb that ground for her. Ice cream bribes, persuasive friends, or obnoxious moves from me won't convince her to continue on a path that's just slightly harder than she thinks she can handle. She has to convince herself she can handle it.

Here's the thing about false flats, though: Once in a while, you turn around and see that the road behind you does, in fact, go downhill and you've actually already made it really far. So far, in this case, she made it through the whole dance, in front of an audience, hands firmly out of her mouth.

As she leapt and tiptoed and rolled, she continued her climb.

12

TRAIL RUNNING: **VENTURING INTO THE WILD**

By Dimity

If George W. was the decider, then I'm the unrememberer. Ask me to recount the plot of any book I've ever I read, and I'm SOL, which is a little shameful for a writer to admit. (What happened to that Russian chick Anna Karenina again?) I've never folded lines from *Caddyshack, Dodgeball,* or some other immensely quotable movie into a conversation, and I rarely get the reference when others do. I suck at recalling people's names, even minutes after being introduced, and have pulled more U-turns in my life than the Dukes of Hazzard.

So it shouldn't come as a surprise when I tell you I can't remember houses I've run past hundreds of times, the turnaround point of a race I've done three times, or how the 14th mile of my last 15-miler felt (which, it should be noted, was almost 3 years ago, so maybe I'm off the hook on that one). Yet I must have selective memory loss, as my sieve-like brain holds onto trail runs for years, almost decades.

Close my eyes, and I can see the dust kicked up by feet stomping on the grayish silt that lines the Central Park Reservoir; the short, steep hills of the Dale Ball Trails in Santa Fe that slowed my pace long after I'd topped them; the brutal 2-mile climb that kicks off the Aspen Golden Leaf Half-Marathon, a trail race, and noodled my legs for the remaining 11.1 miles; the snake-like trails, dotted with bunnies, that wind around Garden of the Gods in Colorado Springs. I can actually picture distinct portions of those runs, which is almost spooky considering I can't recollect the name of any character in *Anna Karenina,* except, of course, ol' Anna herself.

Thinking about it, though, I came to this realization: I use road running—and movies and books—to Calgon me away from my daily life. I put my brain on cruise control and run without thinking about running. But trade smooth pavement for uneven trails and suddenly I'm not tuning

TAKE IT *From* A MOTHER
WHAT'S YOUR FAVORITE TRAIL?

"The ones in Sundance, Utah. They were my first experience with trail running, and it was fabulous!"

—TINA (mantra that fires her up: "Boston, Boston, Boston.")

"None. Trail running requires focus and paying attention, so I haven't tried it yet."

—KAREN (buys new shoes when the old ones start to smell.)

"The Imogene Pass, a 17-mile run from Ouray to Telluride, Colorado. Finishing the race made me feel powerful and deeply fulfilled. It's breathtakingly beautiful and so satisfying to be enjoying that view thanks to my own physical and mental strength."

—LESLIE (quit smoking and started running because she had her eye on a serious cyclist, now her husband.)

"In Kauai, along Poipu Beach, watching whales. But I can find great trails anywhere. I just enjoyed the Lebanon Valley Rail-Trail in Pennsylvania: shaded, flat, and at sea level."

—AMY (usually runs at 6,035 feet above sea level in Colorado Springs.)

"Phoneline Trail in Sabino Canyon in Tucson. It's rugged, steep, and narrow, and the scenery is phenomenal. The Sonoran desert is so alive; as you run, you hear birds chirping and cicadas buzzing, and you see lizards basking in the sun and jackrabbits scurrying about. Due to the difficulty of the trail, it's not heavily traveled. Priceless."

—JESSICA (top three reasons for running: endorphins, it feels like freedom, and it is truly empowering.)

out the world but actually tuning it in. As I ricochet off rocks, hop over roots, and keep track of my route, my brain actively controls the joystick attached to my feet and fires the "jump" and "turbo" buttons endlessly. Like road running, I forget my worry du jour on the dirt—the trails command my attention—but unlike when I'm plodding along on ho-hum streets, I rarely forget the run.

Back up. You're thinking, "Central Park Reservoir is a trail? Really?" OK, my definition is a bit generous there, but in my mind any surface not smoothed out by a yellow machine qualifies as off-road. The perimeter of a golf course works, as do a gravel fire road and, in a pinch, a trodden-down strip of grass next to a sidewalk. In an ideal world, we would all live near narrow, single-track paths that cross bucolic streams and are shaded by aspens. But as adult acne, liverwurst, and other unsavory items attest, the world is far from ideal. Even I, living in a mountainous state overflowing with such trails, can't get to them in the limited window I usually have to run. So I crisscross grassy parks and lope next to train tracks, heeding the oft-repeated mantra in our house: You get what you get, and you don't throw a fit. When I'm not on the pavement, something memorable happens.

Yet as much as I love trails, I don't run on them regularly. In fact, when I'm training for a specific road race, I forgo them completely. Part of it is practical—best to train on the surface you're going to race on so your joints don't get jolted—but part is simply me being way too nerdy. When I've got a detailed training schedule, I can't stand not following it. I want to bull's-eye my mileage and (lickety, 9-minute-mile) pace. Trails typically slow your pace by at least a minute or two (I can't stomach seeing 11-minute-miles when I'm headed to a race) and can also be tricky, footing-wise, for tempo or interval runs. In other words, they don't allow my A+ analness to shine through.

When I cross off my last prescribed workout and cross the finish line on asphalt, though, I'm once again on my trail sabbatical. Getting back on the dirt, I imagine, must be how my kids feel when they run around naked after a bath: totally pure, loving the air on their skin, not worried about what other people think. On the trails, I lose all expectations. I leave the Garmin at home. I usually leave the music at home, too. I run for time—30 minutes, 60 minutes, whatever—but I don't even set my stopwatch on my Timex. I just go off the chronological time, and even then I don't hit the mark because I often have no idea how long a certain loop takes or whether I could've saved time by going left at the last fork. I happily walk when the uphills get too steep, and I don't force it when gravity gifts me on the downhills. The places on my body that scream after a road run barely whisper after a trail run. For good reason: Loamy trails are downright pillowy when compared to unforgiving concrete. Another trail bonus: Useful stabilizing ligaments in ankles and knees, which don't get engaged on the pavement, full-on fire on the trail, building a more bombproof body.

Perhaps most importantly, I live exactly in the moment, not wishing the run away, as I'm prone to do. Prime example: On a recent jaunt in the Garden of the Gods, I, a chronic data checker, didn't even look at my watch until 45 minutes into the run. *No way,* I thought to myself when I finally peeked at it. Yes friggin' way!

My trail runs don't always lead to utopia, though. After a 3-month (real, injury-induced) sabbatical from running, I headed out on a 6-mile hike with the dogs in early January on a Sunday morning, eager to start the New Year right. I had only planned to hike, but after I huffed up the 800-vertical-foot climb at the start, the rest was a gentle downhill. Parts of the trail, hidden from

PRACTICAL *Motherly* ADVICE
BREAD CRUMBS ARE FOR FAIRY TALES

I have no internal navigation, my compass skills are nonexistent, and I couldn't find the North Star if it was the only one in the sky. In short, I'm plum pickings for a wilderness rescue. I get enough drama from my 6-year-old teenager, so here are the no-lose rules I follow:

- I prefer familiar, well-marked trails that have signs with arrows and mileage. Another option is running with a directionally gifted friend or two. I won't go on a new trail by myself unless it feels really established and well-used.

- If I'm by myself on a new trail—a situation into which I rarely put myself—I do an out-and-back, going as straight as possible. If there are forks, I'll go only one direction (like take every left) and only allow myself to take three or so turns before I head back. So when I turn around, I know I take three rights. (Right? Right.)

- On solo runs of any length, I always carry a water bottle and at least one energy gel. (Ballengee had both of those things, plus a shower cap and two ibuprofen.)

- I tell Grant where I'm going and when I expect to be back. (Note: This isn't always foolproof. I tried calling him twice from a helpful stranger's cell phone after my wrist break, and, even though he was home, he didn't pick up either time. "I didn't recognize the number," he explained sheepishly in the ER.)

- On an unfamiliar trail that's a loop, I go with somebody at least twice before I attempt it on my own. The first time, they lead. The second, I lead and don't let them direct me unless I ask for help.

- I'm not afraid to look dumb. Coming down from a hike up a portion of Pike's Peak—read: there's only one direction to go—I noticed a trail I hadn't seen before shoot off the major one. "Is this the main trail down?" I asked a runner zipping past me. "Yep, you've got about 2 miles left," he said. That knowledge made the rest of my run much more enjoyable.

- When in doubt, I head back.

the sun, were slicker than Bill Clinton circa 1998, but long stretches were dirt-covered, open, and just ripe for the running. I couldn't resist. Being uncharacteristically wise, I jogged easily on the clean trails, then stopped and tiptoed across the icy parts. The loop ended in a canyon, which was a veritable ice rink. Stupidly, I kept running; I didn't want my Rocky Mountain high to end. I passed one woman, headed up the canyon, who warned, "Be careful: It's really icy." She's right, I thought, and slowed to a walk. Not a minute later, I was down. Hard, with roughly 90 percent of the impact of my 175-pound body landing directly on my left wrist. It snapped like a dry twig. (Hello, another 3-month sabbatical.)

After I gingerly stood up, sobbing, the first thing I thought to myself was, "Thank God it's just my wrist," as I vaguely remembered a story I had read recently in *Runner's World*. Accomplished adventure racer Danelle Ballengee, who went out for an 8-mile run near her home in Moab, Utah, slid 60 feet down a slick-rock canyon, fractured her pelvis in four places, and survived, in mid-December, for 3 days and 2 nights. Her dog, a 3-year-old named Taz, led rescuers to her. (FYI: I Googled all that info. There was no way my Spongebob mind retained it.) I doubt my hare-brained dogs could've done the same, but I was fortunate to be on a fairly popular trail dotted with people and their fresh New Year's resolutions. Still, I was a bit of a hero. I got back to my standard-transmission truck, loaded up both dogs, and drove home with my knee and right hand, still intact.

Yeah, so the potential for accidents is a big knock against trail running. Unlike road running, when tiny muscle imbalances nibble on you until you're finally injured, you get chomped on the trail: skinned knees, twisted ankles, and broken bones, and you could be miles from your car. Although animal encounters are rare, the annual story of the mountain lion attacking a runner in California always freaks me out. But my biggest fear is getting lost. I haven't yet—knock on wood—but I'm sure that day will come. That said, I'm also fairly confident it'll be a fiasco that lasts an hour or so, nothing longer.

If you've never tried trail running, don't let those last few paragraphs discourage you. If my fairy running-mother appeared one day and told me I had to choose to run exclusively on either trails or the road for the rest of my life, the decision would be a no-brainer: dirt, natch. In fact, as I write this, I've been on a trail extravaganza for about 3 months, and I don't foresee an end date—or a road race—anytime soon. Both my body and mind are thriving. Road running is mostly vanilla, which is America's favorite flavor for a reason: It's reliable and safe and can be easily spruced up with sprinkles and hot fudge or, in this case, intervals or strides. But there are so many more flavors out there. You owe it to yourself to try Rocky Road—with its chunks and surprises packed inside—at least once. It's a taste you won't forget.

.2 THIS IS MY BRAIN ON A RUN
By Dimity

WHAT I THINK ABOUT ON A TYPICAL ROAD RUN

5 percent: Counting the weeks since Grant and I had sex.

5 percent: Imagining how I would feel if I found out I was pregnant again.

5 percent: Contemplating whether I'd want another girl or another boy.

2 percent: There's no chance: It's been 3 weeks since we got busy.

3 percent: Wondering why some (super-hairy, generous-gutted) men think they look good shirtless.

35 percent: Calculating how much time I have left.

10 percent: Convincing myself I do really want to hear "Beautiful Day" by U2 for the bazillionth time.

5 percent: "It's a beautiful day; don't let it get away; it's a beautiful day."

10 percent: Promising myself, for the fiftieth time, I'll make better playlists and delete the tired songs *today*.

3 percent: Planning the (beautiful) day ahead.

2 percent: Remembering a very random date with Maurice, who drove a blue BMW just like that one.

6 percent: Remembering the thank-you notes, already weeks overdue.

8 percent: Visualizing myself with a cold glass of white wine, feet on the coffee table, remote in hand at 8 tonight, telling myself the notes can wait.

0.3 percent: Counting my steps to check my turnover so my stride stays quick and efficient.

0.7 percent: Thinking about my form so I prevent more injuries

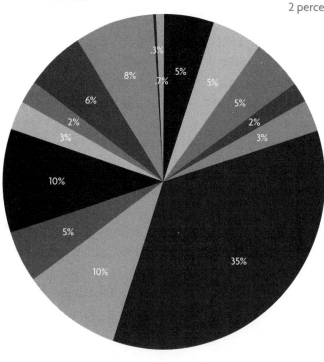

WHAT I THINK ABOUT ON A TYPICAL TRAIL RUN

9 percent: Worrying about a rattlesnake coming out of nowhere and striking my ankle.

17 percent: Convincing myself I'm not lost.

5 percent: Wondering, if I somehow got stranded, who would be the first to notice I was gone.

5 percent: Wondering who would find me. The ideal: a McDreamy EMT.

5 percent: Wondering how long—hours or days?—rescue would take to arrive.

17 percent: Marveling at how much easier trail running feels on my knees and back than road running does.

4 percent: Calculating how much time I have left.

30 percent: Concentrating on where I need to land each foot so I don't twist an ankle.

2 percent: Nothing.

6 percent: Visualizing myself with a cold glass of white wine, feet on the coffee table, remote in hand at 7:30 tonight. Thank-you notes don't even register.

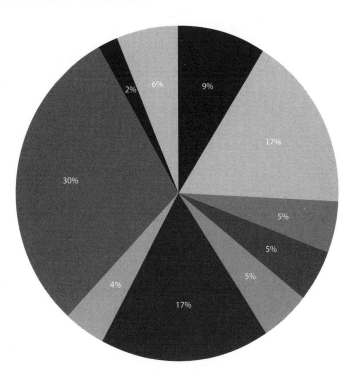

13

CROSS-TRAINING:
SLOWLY STEP AWAY FROM THE ROAD

By Sarah

I had a crappy workout this morning.

It started out dandy; I rode my bike to the outdoor pool. When I got there, I was greeted by a sign saying it was closed for annual cleaning. Irate I'd gotten up too early on a Saturday after an especially demanding workweek, I debated going for a run along the river. But yesterday I did a hard tempo run, and I'm running long tomorrow. I figured my legs needed a rest from the pounding since my left Achilles tendon has been speaking up lately.

So I pedaled to my gym and hopped on a stationary bike for 30 minutes. (I wasn't wearing padded bike shorts, or I would have stayed outside to ride.) Then I did 10 minutes on the elliptical and threw in 5 minutes of core. To me, cardio machines feel like busywork from a substitute teacher instead of an assignment from a demanding taskmaster. I hadn't gotten in a good sweat, and I felt I hadn't accrued any real fitness gains. As I rode home to face the clamoring crowd, I was peeved. Not good: To be in full-time mommy mode on the weekends, I need to feel content after my workouts, not like a malcontent.

Once I got over myself, I started thinking about which cross-training activity best serves my running or gives my tender Achilles tendon or tight hip flexor a break. Experts no longer insist runners cross-train to prevent injury, but after several days on the road, I feel like my 43-year-old body would like a less jarring form of exercise. My mind could use a break too. Here's a rundown of options to help you decide which activity to choose the next time you opt to not hit the road, track, trail, or treadmill—or when you get shut out of the pool.

CYCLING OR SPINNING

What It Works: Quadriceps, glutes, and calf muscles, mainly.

The Good: As Dimity can attest, cycling hard can give a runner explosive power by strengthening the big muscles of the lower body. A nonimpact activity, cycling can provide the same aerobic buck as running without all the bang-bang-bang. It's also fun to be able to cover a lot more ground than you can on foot: What *does* that paved trail look like beyond your usual 5-mile turnaround spot? And the social aspect of spinning is a nice break from the often lonely life of a runner. If you're in your basement, with your bike hooked up to an indoor trainer, you can catch up on the last 5 years of movies or TV shows everybody talks about but you've never seen. (*Who are these* Mad Men *everyone keeps talking about?*)

The Bad: You have to ride hard to stay fit. Tootling around on your bike (or at the gym on a stationary bike) is fine for a recovery day to get the blood moving, but researchers have found you have to pedal intensely enough to get your heart rate up to 80 percent max to enjoy the same cardio-enhancing benefits as running. (Keep your pedals spinning at about ninety revolutions per minute to mimic an ideal running cadence, and wear a heart rate monitor to keep yourself honest.) Oh, and falling on hard pavement or a rocky trail can sideline your running, not to mention your life.

And the Ugly: A butt not used to sitting on a cycling seat is a butt that will be sore for days after your first (and second and third) ride.

SWIMMING

What It Works: Whole body, but especially the back, arms, and core. (You only need to stare at— uh, I mean, *look* at—Michael Phelps's physique to realize swimming hits ab muscles hard!)

The Good: Swimming taxes runners' oft-neglected upper body while giving their overworked lower bodies a break. Doing various strokes takes some skill, which engages the brain. It's delightful to be in a cool, wet environment and to be horizontal. Pool running is an adequate option for injured or pregnant runners. (In the later months of my pregnancy with Phoebe, I strapped a foam belt around my big ol' belly and hit the deep end about twice a week.)

The Bad: Proficiency is an issue; if you didn't learn to swim as a kid, be prepared to flail, and then find time to take lessons. Finding a nearby pool with convenient lap times and uncrowded lanes can also be a challenge. As for pool running, even the most hip-happening playlist in the world couldn't

TAKE IT *From* A MOTHER
WHAT'S YOUR BEST CROSS-TRAINING WORKOUT?

"I like to swim because it's excellent recovery from the hard pounding my legs take from running. Plus, it hits muscles that don't get worked from running and lets my legs mend their soreness."

—JILL (top three reasons for running: to make a bad day good, to clear my head, and to make myself a better me.)

"In Zumba, a dance-inspired aerobics class, I get to shake my hips, feel the rhythm of great Latin tunes, and remember dance steps. The downside is some of the moves that twist and turn can be hard on the knees."

—JEANETTE (also likes to walk shelter dogs at the Humane Society.)

"Spinning. I had calf issues with my first marathon. I started taking spinning classes three times a week after the race. A few months later, when I ran my second marathon, I had no calf problems at all. The classes really helped to balance out my legs."

—AMANDA (dream place to run: The Great Wall.)

"My favorite X-training workout is aqua jogging because I can get a total body workout in my pool. By the time I get out, I feel like a piece of spaghetti without feeling like I've impacted my muscles in an adverse way."

—MARY (worst part of running: "when I plan to run but then can't.")

"Yoga, without a doubt. I love it and would do it every day if I had the time. When I go on a regular basis, I feel very strong."

—TRYNA (vowed to run a marathon when she was on modified bed rest while pregnant with twins.)

"I love to kayak. It's a great change of pace, a wonderful way to be outdoors, and it's quite a core workout."

—JENNIFER (doesn't trust race spectators who tell her she's almost there.)

"Sadly, I don't cross train."

—AMY (longest distance ever run: 26.2 miles. "I don't plan on going any farther.")

make pool running fun for me. And unless you have a waterproof carrier, listening to tunes while swimming isn't an option.

And the Ugly: Chlorine is an evil chemical. Yes, it counteracts leakage from swim diapers, but it also turns your skin to leather and your hair to straw.

ELLIPTICAL

What It Works: Primarily the legs and glutes, with a smattering of arms and back thrown in if you use a machine with movable, pole-like handles.

The Good: Since your feet never leave the pedals, tracing oval circles on the elliptical gives your joints a free ride, avoiding the impact of running. Good for training while healing an injury, if pedaling doesn't aggravate it. You can easily vary the intensity and incline and add in the upper body for some variation. It's indoors—yet not the treadmill—so a *People* from 6 months ago can take your mind off the tedium.

The Bad: As on the bike, you've got to focus on intensity or you'll have nothing more than a nice recovery workout. I rarely see anyone at my gym going hard enough on an elliptical to mimic running. Also, the length of the strides is usually pre-set, which means if you're unusually short or tall, you'll feel unbalanced.

And the Ugly: Klutzy runners, me included, can find the motion awkward, especially trying to change direction and push the pedals in reverse. (While working out, I have so much leg strength yet so little brain power.)

ROWING OR ROWING MACHINE (AKA ERGOMETER OR "ERG")

What It Works: Pretty much everything, from shoulders, back, and core down to glutes and legs.

The Good: Aerobically challenging, rowing is a low-impact workout that demands equal parts concentration and technique. In the gym, when you're rowing correctly, an erg rivals the Gauntlet (the stairclimber with stairs, not pedals) and the VersaClimber (the vertical pole with pedals) for the most demanding and underused cardio machine. To nail your form, ask a trainer, or better yet, a rower who looks like she knows what she's doing. A quick hint: Extend your legs, swing your torso back, pull your arms toward you, then extend your arms, lean forward, fold your legs. Plus, you gotta love a sport where you can sit down *and* go backward toward the finish line. Or at least I definitely do.

Run LIKE THIS MOTHER
A VARIATION TO TRI

By Dimity

For all a triathlete's talk about dialed-in carbon fiber bike frames, smooth transition tactics—switching from swimming to biking and then from biking to running—and other intimidating posturing, here's a secret: Triathlons are actually easier, in many ways, than pure running races. Instead of doing one joint-pounding motion again and again and mentally berating yourself to pound harder and faster, you get to switch up the muscles you use and the way you use them three times, making both the physical effort and mental focus much easier.

First you swim. The start can be helter-skelter, with limbs flying everywhere, and even I, a pretty capable swimmer, often drink more lake water than recommended. So before your first tri—I'd recommend starting with a sprint length, which is a 750-meter (less than half a mile) swim, a 12-ish mile bike, and a 5K run—you may need a few swim lessons. You'll also probably want to rent a wetsuit, which makes you more buoyant and eases the effort of your swim. Swimming uses predominantly your upper body, keeping your legs fresh for the rest of the race. (If the swim still stops you from considering a triathlon, know that plenty of people swim backstroke or breaststroke for a stretch—or the entire race. Total fish out of water? Opt for a bike–run duathlon.)

Then you get out of the water, slither out of your wetsuit, and hop on the bike. My best, most anticipated athletic rush is the first few miles of the bike in a triathlon on a sunny day. Chilly and wet from the swim, you get goose bumps from the wind breezing by you on the bike, making your muscles feel fresh, fast, and powerful. Within a few miles, you're fairly dry and are simply pushing your legs around in circles. It's the most peaceful part of the race: There's no impact on your body, you get a chance to recover when you hit a downhill, and cycling has that helpful element of momentum. For your first tri, a mountain bike with slick road tires, or even a hybrid bike, is totally fine.

Then you hit the run. (I know you have running shoes, so don't try to argue with me there.) Your legs definitely feel drained, and your energy level isn't the same as it is when you start a 5K fresh, but you've still got something to work with: You're familiar with the sport. So you take off, and you curse and hate me for suggesting you do this. Then, somehow, your legs snap back and you're chugging along, riding on the high that the race is two thirds over. You've only got 3 little miles to go? Cake.

Back at the transition area, energized and unbelievably proud, you find yourself clandestinely checking out the carbon fiber frames and contemplating a purchase of your own. Another triathlete is born.

The Bad: First, there's the water thing: Arizonians probably don't have rowing as an option. Takes skill and experience to get in a boat; it's hard, but not impossible, to pick up the sport as an adult. If you do find a program, you usually need at least one other person, if not a minivan full of other rowers, to take out a boat.

And the Ugly: If you row outside, be prepared for blisters on your palms so severe, you'll shriek when the shower-water hits them.

WALKING
What It Works: Legs and butt, mainly.

The Good: Walking is far less joint-jarring than our friend running: A walker hits the ground with only the force of her body weight, whereas a runner lands with up to three times that. The slower pace of walking lets you take in the scenery (or stop and snoop over a neighbor's fence or peek in a store window).

The Bad: If weight loss or management is your aim, you need to spend a lot more time walking than running to get the same outcome. No matter how you cover a route—ambling or sprinting—you burn roughly 100 calories per mile. So if you want to incinerate 300 calories, you can either run for about a half hour or walk for about 45 minutes.

And the Ugly: Let's just be honest: Walking doesn't have the same hip, sexy factor as running does.

YOGA
What It Works: Flexibility, strength, and balance.

The Good: An unbeatable stress reliever, yoga also releases muscle tightness, increases range of motion, and enhances balance. Yogic breathwork translates into breath control while running, which, with time, can also translate into a more efficient stride. Some yoginis claim it calms mind-monkeys even better than running. Good way to challenge yourself in a non–speed-oriented way: headstand without the wall, anyone?

The Bad: It's hard to knock this activity—Lord knows what doing so will do to my karma—but to this runner who loves motion, I find it d-u-l-l. I feel great after class, but during it, time creeps by.

And the Ugly: Being surrounded by hyper-flexible reeds, touching their foreheads to the ground while bent over with straight knees, makes me feel like a rigid board.

PILATES

What It Works: Your core, baby!

The Good: Whether done on a mat in a class setting or individually on a Reformer contraption, Pilates corrects running-induced imbalances such as too many miles on a canted road or with incorrect form. Repeated core work gives you strength you thought you'd never regain after a C-section. Lots of hip exercises provide welcome relief of tightness and restore mobility in this overworked joint.

The Bad: Classes can run you $15 or more: Do I invest in a six-pack of classes or a new pair of running shoes?

And the Ugly: Running makes you think you're super fit, but a set of Teasers on a Box later, your abs quivering, and you're not so sure.

.2 MY RUNNING NEUROSIS
By Sarah

You say Powerade, I say Gatorade. Even though we runners are one united, chafed group, every runner has her tics. In order to make you feel less concerned about yours (really? You stop your watch at every. single. stoplight?), here are some of mine:

- I always put on my right running shoe first, figuring I need to put my best foot (aka my "right" foot, not my "wrong" foot) forward.

- I believe my iPod sends me a subliminal message, via the first song it plays, about my upcoming run. I then spend the first half-mile or so trying to decipher what the message is. Lenny Kravitz's "Dig In" is a gimme, but the B-52s' "Funplex" is more cryptic.

- I always have to finish my run at a crack in the middle of our driveway. No matter how long the run or how drag-ass I feel, I force myself to that exact spot before slowing to a walk.

- I run outside year-round, no matter what the weather gods throw at me. And I don tights only when it's 20 degrees or colder. Otherwise I sport capris or a running skirt.

- If I'm wearing my Brooks Vapor Dry 2 gloves, I take them off and snap the magnet-laden wrists together exactly one half-block from my house.

- I run on the road in almost every situation: I have to be facing down a bus with a garbage truck barreling up behind me to hop onto the sidewalk.

- My idea of Shangri-La is the Hood to Coast, a 196-mile relay that involves being trapped in an increasingly stinky van with five other runners, hopping out in the middle of nowhere along Oregon backroads to run at random hours of the day *and* night, and getting by on catnaps for about 28 hours. No 3G service, no showers, no flush toilets, no space to stretch cramping legs.
I love every bit of it.

- I go through a short stint of depression at the start of daylight savings time. I should be psyched for BBQs in long-lasting sunlight or after-work tennis matches, but the time switch means I'm back to dark morning runs for at least another month.

- I contemplate going for a run on a glorious spring day when I spot someone running in the afternoon—even when I've already logged five miles that morning.

14

STRENGTH TRAINING: **PUT SOME MUSCLE INTO IT**

By Dimity

Once, while on spring break in Florida, I went to the grocery store with my very opinionated grand-mother. In the Publix parking lot, a red sports car darted in front of her light blue Chevy wagon, causing her to slam on the brakes.

She didn't miss a beat. "Never trust anyone, Dimmy, who drives a little red sports car," she said, tapping her finger forcefully on the pleather steering wheel cover. "They're always bad news."

Questionable advice, for sure, but it's stuck with me. I'm now oddly suspicious of drivers of tiny red cars. I also have a hard time naturally trusting

- Really overweight doctors (a few extra pounds, fine; they work stressful hours, and hospital cafeterias make elementary school lunchrooms seem like five-star restaurants)

- Any woman who, within 5 minutes of our first meeting, details her sex life

- Celebrities who hawk wares on the Home Shopping Channel

- People who shop at Christmas stores that are open year-round

- Fitness writers who don't stretch, strength train, do yoga or Pilates, or otherwise embrace a well-rounded routine

I was firmly in that last group for more than a decade. Sure, in my sleep I could list reasons why you should strength train—a sleeker bod, injury prevention, stronger bones, better metabolism—as surely as I can robotically write up a total-body toning routine that, as guaranteed in the story introduction, helps you lose 10 pounds in just 6 weeks! But had I ever followed a magazine workout? Nope. Not once. Occasionally,

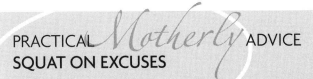

PRACTICAL *Motherly* ADVICE
SQUAT ON EXCUSES

Women's magazines like to throw in the occasional television workout, advising readers to do squats, lunges, or planks during the commercials. I think I'd have better luck winning the Boston Marathon than motivating off the couch when I'm vegging. But, hey, if it works for you, I'm beyond impressed. If not, some other ideas to squeeze it in:

9 Cut a weekly run or two short by 15 minutes and strength train instead. If it's a nice day, do it in a park or a friendly neighbor's yard so you're not at home. A body weight routine of squats, lunges, planks, sit-ups, and push-ups is more than enough to fill your strength RDA.

9 Do a wall-sit as you brush your teeth.

9 "Run 20 minutes to the gym, 20 minutes of strength training, 20 minutes back."

—MARY (feels strongest when doing pull-ups.)

9 "If I'm playing on the floor with my baby daughter, I do sit-ups, push-ups, and leg lifts and use her as a weight while I'm down there. I often get more done in a day than I may have if I tried to do a straight 15-minute core routine."

—SARI (dream running date: a trail run followed by a milkshake and a shower.)

9 "I have a rule of 10 for my upper body: I tell myself, if I can just get in 10 triceps dips or push-ups, I'll have met my quota for the day. But it's really a trick because if I can do 10, chances are quite high I'll do 10 reps of another exercise. I do the same thing with abs, but that number is 25."

—MARY (swears by glucosamine chondroitin supplements for her joints.)

I'd be forced to do a half-hearted run-through of a routine to gauge its difficulty or figure out how long it took, but it ended there. I liked my exercise straight-up and sweaty: running, preferably, but I'd also take a StairMaster, spinning class, or stationary bike. The sign of a good workout was a sports bra I had to wring out immediately in the locker room, not triceps that were tender to the touch 48 hours after the workout.

That instant gratification mentality began to erode after I had my second kid. At the end of the day, I regularly noticed the indent of my belt on my "abs," which oozed over my jeans like a melting ice cream cone. Every time I had to squeeze into a pair of dress pants—not often, thank goodness—I

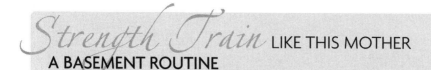

Strength Train LIKE THIS MOTHER
A BASEMENT ROUTINE

When your kids are watching TV—oops, I mean quietly doing art projects, practicing their Spanish flashcards, or cleaning their rooms—get busy and mix-and-match with this list of ingredients. I do two sets of twelve to fifteen reps of eight various exercises, alternating between upper and lower body with minimal rest. For example: squat, plank, squat, plank, lunge, triceps, lunge, triceps, and so on.

LOWER BODY
Squats Two Ways

ONE LEGGED: Stand, on one foot, near a wall or stair railing for balance. Slowly bend that knee, going no lower than 45 degrees and keeping your knee in line with your ankle.

WALL SITS: Back against the wall, knees 90 degrees, hold. Running goddess Kathrine Switzer, in her book *Marathon Woman,* said it was the best exercise she knew to prevent knee pain. She took it to the extreme, building up to 11 minutes, but a goal of 2 minutes works for me.

Step-Ups

Step up slooooowly with one foot onto a step until your standing leg is straight. Lower slowly and start again. If your muscles aren't burning by the fifteenth rep, you're going too fast.

Lunges

Rest your back leg on a stability ball, bend your front knee, then straighten.

Crab Walk

Put an exercise band around both ankles, then squat down to about 30 degrees, and step sideways across the floor. Builds the gluteus medius, a really important (and neglected) stabilizing muscle.

UPPER BODY AND CORE
Back Extensions

Two choices. On a stability ball: Rest your knees or toes on the floor and your stomach on the ball, and lift your back. Or on the floor: Lie on your stomach and raise arms and legs at the same time, like Superman.

Plank

Rest on elbows and toes, back straight, butt down. My fave: It's like running fast. Super hard, but over quickly and very effective.

Side Planks

Rest on left elbow, outer side of left foot, right foot stacked on left foot.

Crunches

Contract your abs on a stability ball, on the floor, like you're riding a bike, twisting side to side—the options are endless.

Triceps Dips

Rest your palms, fingers facing out, on a chair or table, with your legs straight, heels on the floor. Bend your elbows straight back, then push up.

Push-Ups

A few options, going from easiest to hardest:

- Hands on the stairs, like the fourth one from the ground. With time, go one step lower.

- Knees on floor.

- Knees on stability ball.

- Shins on stability ball.

- Real ones: toes and palms on the floor.

- Feet on the stability ball. (If you can do 10 in a row, you're my hero.)

had to resurrect the life-sucking girdle-y thing I wore on my wedding day. My lower back, never one to edit its pain, was tender to the touch, but not from any workout.

So I staged my own intervention. With the marathon story assignment, Sarah and I were fortunate enough to be given coaches. I told Ivana, my coach, that besides crossing the finish line with pride and limbs intact, my next priority was getting strong. Or, as I have explained in countless magazine stories, I would have a hard time going the distance.

Here's why: The core, an area that runs from the bottom of your ribs to the bottom of your bum, is the metaphorical mother of your body. Her strength dictates your overall strength. If she's weak and loosey-goosey, there is no discipline in your body. Your legs overstride, your arms splay like a sprinkler, and you'll probably end up injured (or at least frustrated because you never get faster). If she keeps a tight ship and barks out multiple orders at once—instructing your feet to turn over quickly and lightly, your lower back muscles to stabilize, your arms to swing tightly—the better runner you'll be. If she has to focus on one weak part of the body, like your right hip, bribing it with TLC so it will move along, some other part, like your left glute, will disobey and flare up. The situation is not unlike bribing an ornery 3-year-old with fruit snacks, who tells an otherwise content 6-year-old that it was the last pack, who then throws a fit.

Two babies out, I needed a happy, solid core that would support the distance (and I definitely didn't mind the idea of being a bit sleeker). My routine for the marathon was very simple: six to eight exercises that required either a stability ball or only body weight and therefore could be done at home.

I lied. The routine itself was simple; getting it done was anything but. A 20-minute strength routine, interrupted by Amelia asking for a chocolate chip cookie at 7:20 A.M. and Ben thinking pulling every book in the bookcase is a grand game, took more than 45 minutes. I was supposed to do the routine 3 days a week. I averaged twice and sometimes only got to it once. But even my C+ effort paid off significantly. My lower back became less achy. My stomach, while far from a six-pack, at least stopped being tattooed daily by my belt. Lifting and carrying my tugboats—I mean children—didn't feel like such a chore. Overall, I felt much more stable and capable, like my limbs could actually work as a team, not free agents.

But then, after my marathon, I retired the planks. I was burnt out on basement routines and training in general. I soon discovered that was a big mistake, as I was quickly back to an aching back and sloppy abs. Which is something I pretty much hate about exercise: It has no savings account. You either make regular deposits in the strength and cardiovascular accounts, or your balance quickly falls to zero. Sure, it's easier to regain strength and aerobic fitness if your muscles already know the drill, but anything more than a week or two off, and your body pulls the "who-me?" act, commonly seen in children asked to do chores: They moan and groan and pretend they can't remember how it's done.

But if you're like me, in your late thirties, this is no time to baby your body. As far as strength training goes, it's do-or-die time. According to Wayne Westcott, Ph.D., a senior fitness executive at the South Shore YMCA in Massachusetts and exercise science wizard, you lose, on average, 6 pounds of muscle every decade of adult life. Lean muscle is the worker bee of your metabolic system: It burns

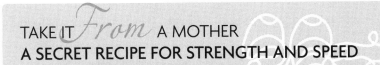

TAKE IT *From* A MOTHER
A SECRET RECIPE FOR STRENGTH AND SPEED

Kerrie and Kat's strength and cardio combo is a workout worthy of a magazine cover line: "Get Stronger and Faster Now!" "The lifting seems like it would be easy, but then you throw in sprints and, all of a sudden, twenty-four body-weight squats are rather fatiguing," says Kat. Adds trainer Kerrie, "The circuits, combined with fast running, mimics the demands of a marathon, when you have to keep running despite increasing weariness."

Warm up with a 2-mile jog on a treadmill.

Run 400 meters at 5K pace.

Twelve burpees (from a standing position, jump feet back to push-up position, jump feet forward, repeat).

Six assisted chin-ups.

Thirty crunches.

Twelve push-ups.

Twenty-four body-weight squats (hold a medicine ball if you want).

Run 400 meters.

Ten squats with shoulder press.

Eight push-ups with feet, shins, or knees on stability ball.

Twelve triceps dips.

Thirty back extensions.

Thirty lunges with biceps curls.

Repeat once, then cool down with, as Kat says, "whatever energy you have left."

calories all the time, and revs up during and after strength workouts. The more muscle you have, the faster your body processes the grilled cheese crusts you ate for lunch. And muscle also supports your bones and posture, which, as I know from spending too much time in Publix stores, can wither with age, leaving old ladies, struck with osteoporosis, hunched and forever staring at their Velcro sneakers. Unfortunately, running alone doesn't build muscle; in fact, says Westcott, a decade-long University of Florida study on master's runners found they lost 5 pounds of muscle in 10 years.

Find time to squeeze in 20 minutes two or three times a week, and I promise it will make a difference in your running, your health, your daily life. But in case I've branded myself as a little red sports car driver in your mind, don't take my advice. "I've trained for races without weight training and then I trained for racing using weight circuits," says Kerrie, a personal trainer who has four kids (and still, ahem, finds time to weight train). "There was no comparison." Back in the day, Kerrie trained Kat, a mother of two, for a half-marathon, the only race Kat has run injury-free.

"When I slack off of weights, I am slower and more sluggish and heavier," says Kat, who is not being paid for this appearance. "I actually lose weight when I strength train." There's an endorsement way more believable than any Jessica Simpson has done for acne medication.

.2 A FEW OF MY FAVORITE THINGS
By Dimity

Julie Andrews might have gone for snowflakes that stay on her nose and eyelashes, but I like

9 Running in the rain.

9 Napping midday after a long run. (Full disclosure: I park the kids, with a snack, in front of a video and say, "Don't bug me for anything.")

9 Holding Warrior I and II poses in yoga, which stretch out my inner thighs and, in doing so, seem to unkink the rest of my lower body.

9 Deflating a blister under an angry toenail. I get the point of a safety pin really hot with a match, jab it under (or through) the nail, then squeeze out the blood and gunk until there's nothing left. Yuck, but aahhh.

9 Coasting on a slight downhill.

9 Slipping on a dry shirt after a long run or race for the drive home. (Assuming, of course, I remember to bring one.)

9 Doing a new race instead of a familiar one a second time.

9 Reminding myself, at mile 10 of a 14-miler, that tomorrow is a day off.

9 Sporting a race T-shirt that is actually cute and actually fits. (In the fifty or so races I've done in my life, only one falls into that category.)

9 Reveling in the first chilly fall run, when I don't need to shed my long-sleeve top, and again in the first spring one, when long sleeve is finally not necessary.

9 Playing hooky in the middle of a long training cycle. Instead of pulling on my sports bra and tights, I get naked and spend the length of time I would've been running in the bathroom. I put a clay mask on my face and slide into a hot bubble bath, Epsom salts optional. I read a chapter or two of my book before meticulously shaving my legs and attacking my calluses with a pumice stone. When I get out, I tweeze the witch hairs on my face, clip my toenails, and apply lotion.

9 Reading the race listings in the back of magazines.

9 Remembering to heed, just as I'm about to launch into an internal you're-so-slow diatribe, the advice my coach Abby gave me: "Don't say anything to yourself you wouldn't say to a friend."

15

NUTRITION: CARB-O-NATION

By Sarah

As much as I love my husband and kids, what I really live for are carbohydrates. Pasta, bagels, oatmeal, rice, pizza, more pasta. Ergo, I was the ideal guinea pig for *Runner's World* to put on the popular low-carb South Beach Diet for 2 weeks to see how I'd fare. I was game: I wanted to look like I exercise as frequently as I do, not as my belly pouch incorrectly suggests. Plus, I was intrigued to see what the protein-dense, carb-starved diet would do to my energy level.

What's so special about carbs? They're a quick and easy source of glucose, the sugar present in your blood, muscles, and liver. To function, your body needs glucose or glycogen, which is what glucose is called when it's stored in your muscles and liver. Your brain and nerves rely exclusively on glucose to keep humming, but the two don't have any storage capacity, so they always access the blood for sugar. (This is why when your blood sugar drops in a race or long run, you feel more pain, and your thoughts turn negative. As in, *Why do I do this dumb sport?*) Meanwhile, muscles burn a mix of glucose and fat for fuel. The more intense the session (speed) or the more strength needed (hills), the richer that mix is in glucose. At sprint speeds, for instance, 100 percent of your energy is derived from carbohydrates.

The bottom line: Skimp on carbs, and your body can quickly run out of fuel.

Carbs, schmarbs. Who needed them? I stocked up on chicken, fish, eggs, low-fat cheeses, nuts, and veggies. On a sun-dappled Monday, I embarked on a carb-free experiment. It's not one I'd recommend repeating.

DAY 1

My first low-carb meal of scrambled eggs with low-fat cheese and a small glass of V-8 juice leaves me feeling empty on my trail run with my then-2-year-old daughter, Phoebe, whose omnipresent bag of Goldfish taunts me the entire way.

DAY 3

Midway through an easy 5-mile run with my new friend, Ellison, my quads feel tapped, and I have to plead for a walking break. For the rest of the evening, I'm depleted; I've felt perkier after 18-mile training runs.

DAY 5

Whoever said fish is brain food was wrong: Jack, who joined me on diet in show of solidarity, and I agree this diet is making us stupid and forgetful. I eat surprisingly tasty homemade black bean soup (the recipe is in *The South Beach Diet Cookbook*) for lunch. A mere four servings of it finally satisfies me.

DAY 10

On a run 2 days ago, I never shook the once-I-get-warmed-up-I'll-be-fine feeling in my quads. I huffed and puffed so loudly, I could barely hear the birds singing. And today my thighs strain to keep the pedals moving on the elliptical.

DAY 11

In Pilates, after 25 minutes of cardio machines, I bottom out. I get lightheaded and disoriented doing hundreds, and I can only do about half the reps of all the moves. My muscles—and my mind—are miserable.

DAY 14

What a way to end this diet: with halibut on a simple bed of wild rice, lentils, and a single serving of basmati rice. I feel my engine start to rev a bit higher as I put in its regular octane.

Like many low-carb dieters, I lost about 8 pounds in 2 weeks. Probably because of the lack of bread, but also because my dessert cravings seemed weaker than before. Yet a few days later, my appetite for Trader Joe's Way More Chocolate Chips Cookies came roaring back. Ten days after that, my eating habits reverted basically back to my version of normal. And the rest of me was, thankfully,

TAKE IT *From* A MOTHER
WHAT'S YOUR FAVORITE PRE-RUN FUEL?

"It used to be a Payday candy bar. Now it's Gatorade."

—AMY (strength train? "Does carrying 20-pound twins count?")

"Oatmeal and a scrambled egg if it's the morning. Midday, I go for rice with chicken or turkey—and hot sauce. Yum!"

—SUSAN (before a marathon: does four 23- to 24-mile runs.)

"Nothing usually."

—KATHY (ran first marathon to impress her then-boyfriend, now husband.)

"Any sports bar containing chocolate and peanut butter, and coffee."

—JULIE (listens to music while strength training to avoid socializers who eat up time.)

"Avocado."

—DANA (started running because a boyfriend (falsely) said she couldn't run a 10K as fast as he could.)

"Oatmeal and a fruit-and-yogurt smoothie."

—JENNIFER (has nursed on the side of a road during a run. "Trying to get my boob back into the sweaty sports bra is always interesting.")

"When running in the A.M. I load up on oatmeal, banana, toast with peanut butter, sometimes a red potato, and water."

—DEBBIE (has been a runner for 40 years.)

"Toast topped with steamed spinach and an egg white. Or a piece of Laffy Taffy if I'm feeling sluggish. Sometimes I need a sugar spike to get me going."

—JUNKO (post-run meal: any leftovers in the fridge. "I'm not picky.")

"I'm a peanut-butter-and-honey-on-toast girl."

—LESLIE (overtrained, "I am not nice and very teary.")

"I am still trying to figure this one out."

—RUTH ANNE (favorite post-run snack: Granny Smith apple, cut up, dipped in peanut butter and homemade granola.)

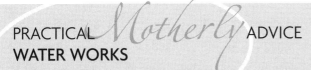

PRACTICAL *Motherly* ADVICE
WATER WORKS

On long marathon training runs, unless you're a 7-minute miler or 100-ish pounds, you probably need to drink more than you can carry. A couple of ideas to keep your post-run pee as pale as when you set out:

- Stash a bottle (or two) under a tree at a midway point of your run. (Freeze it the night before, so it'll still be cold when you pick it up 2 hours into your long run.)

- Make the water chilly, flavored, and salty. Research shows athletes chug-a-lug more when beverages are cool, have flavor, and include the electrolyte sodium.

- Create a route so you'll run by a friend's or your house for a refill. (Have an assistant waiting outside for the hand-off: Nothing kills momentum on a long run faster than a prolonged, inert stop.)

- Plan a route that includes some parks with water fountains.

- Carry a couple bucks and treat yourself to a Gatorade at a gas station. (In a pinch, I've also filled up my bottle in a gas station sink bathroom in New York City. Not recommended.)

- Recruit a pal (or your husband) to pedal next to you, toting refreshments. It doesn't have to be the final miles of your run; they can caddy for you for several miles, then give you a full bottle before they depart.

too. Three days post-diet, Ellison and I ran the same route we did on Day 3, and I was peppy and chatty for all 5 miles. A month post-diet, and I'm pretty sure I regained those 8 pounds.

I now look back on those 2 weeks with utter horror: I've rarely felt so miserable. Despite its name, V-8 is not fuel for running. Many interviews with sports nutritionists later, I know what a bad, *bad* idea a limited-carbohydrate diet is for a runner. Yet there's no reason to swing hard in the other direction and become a pasta-eating machine. I've cut way back on my bagel consumption, and I no longer drink OJ every morning.

What you eat and drink depends on the distance or the amount of time you're running. Here's a look at nutrition before, during, and after a run.

PRACTICAL *Motherly* ADVICE
GRAB-AND-GO FUEL

My rowing teammate Marcie recently found a vintage chocolate PowerBar, circa 1997, buried in her glove compartment. For kicks, we ripped it open and took a bite. (Hey, before an early morning workout, everything seems a whole lot funnier.) I could almost still taste the chocolate, and it made me think of the days when a PowerBar was the only on-the-go energy option. Now the sports nutrition aisle rivals the cereal one at most supermarkets, with the choices falling into three main categories:

BARS

THE SKINNY: An easy, ever-ready option before or after a run. Hard to eat while running, though. But great for triathletes because the bar, unwrapped, sticks right on a bike frame. New flavors and formulations make them infinitely more palatable than their last-millennium predecessors.

FAVES: PowerBar Energize, Luna Bar, Clif Bar, Larabars.

GELS

THE SKINNY: A quick blast of 100 calories that needs no chewing. Consistency is like runny icing. Can be hard to gag down the first few times. (Insert tasteless "spit-or-swallow" comment here.) Easy absorption in your blood provides almost instant energy. Available with or without caffeine or extra sodium. Empty wrappers are sticky, so best to eat one near a trash can.

FAVES: GU Sports Gel, PowerBar Gel, Clif Shot.

CHEWS

THE SKINNY: Gummi candies for grown-ups. Open before you run, stuff a few in your pocket, and eat just what you want; nibble a lot or a little. Can be a nice distraction to work one around your mouth for a half-mile or so—and then spend the next mile or so picking bits of it out of your teeth.

FAVES: Clif Shot Bloks, Sport Beans, PowerBar Gel Blasts, GU Chomps.

WHAT TO EAT AND DRINK BEFORE

If you are headed out on a typical 30- to 45-minute weekday run, you don't need to put anything more than water into your body before you hit the road. Even if you're running first thing, your body has enough energy stored to power you through your workout. How much water you glug depends on how thirsty you feel and when you last drank. For a morning runner who has gone all night with nothing more than a midnight sip after soothing her preschooler back to sleep, it's a good idea to drink at least 8 ounces of water before heading out the door. But if you're running on your lunch break or after putting the kids to bed, the leading experts advise runners to "drink to thirst." Which means drink normally through the day, when you feel like it, and drink some water before heading out if you feel the need. Personally, I sweat buckets, so I drink at least 16 ounces of *agua* before a 5-mile run. If you're a runner who has to have a pre-run coffee, stop beating yourself up about it: A cup of joe may help you. (Studies have shown that caffeine can help an athlete run longer *and* make the work feel easier.)

As you get closer to running for an hour, though, you've got to ramp up your calories a bit. Beforehand, take a few swigs of a sports drink or juice, or eat a small piece of fruit, like a banana, along with a glass of water. If you're going longer than 90 minutes, try to eat a small, balanced meal before the run. Ideas: a bowl of cereal topped with berries and milk, half a turkey sandwich on whole-grain bread, or a grilled cheese sandwich. Even if you think you'll get leaner if you skimp on calories, you're going to conk out or turn around sooner instead of going strong. Depending on your stomach, your meal can be eaten as long as 2 hours before or right before you slip on your Mizunos.

Experiment with what works with you. I eat a bowl of steel-cut oats mixed with nuts and yogurt immediately before my runs, and my stomach feels fine before all my double-digit runs, whereas Julie, an occasional running buddy, has a very sensitive digestive system and often has to make emergency pit stops when she eats anything solid. Through a process of trial and error and porta-potty stops, she's found her tummy can tolerate a smoothie made of yogurt, frozen blueberries, half of a banana, and a small scoop of whey protein before a long run. When she drinks the concoction an hour before the run, she can run worry-free.

WHAT TO EAT AND DRINK DURING

On a run that's about 75 minutes or less, there's no need to haul any extra calories; you can rely on the energy (aka glycogen) stored in your muscles and the food you eat beforehand to carry you through. Let your thirst level and the weather dictate whether you carry water with you. Living in a cool and moist (some would say "rainy") climate like Portland, I opt to go empty handed, but in arid Denver, Dimity totes a bottle on warmer days. One caveat: When you are running at high intensities (such as interval workouts) for about an hour, taking in carbohydrate and fluid can improve the quality of your effort.

Run longer, however, and you need to take in about 60 grams of carbohydrates every hour (a single gram of carbs has 4 calories, so that's about 240 calories), along with fluid. Those carbs can come from many sources, but the two most common are sports drinks and energy gels. Sports nutritionists are quick to point out that gels and sports drinks are sugar by another name. The white stuff is what your body wants when it's in motion for an extended period of time, so feel free to chomp on gummi bears, Tootsie Rolls, dried fruit, or Twizzlers if they're more appealing. I know a sports nutritionist, a veteran of nine marathons, who indulges in Milky Ways on her long runs, and another one who nibbles Fig Newtons and Oreos.

But don't pay an impromptu visit to Dairy Queen for a Blizzard at mile 12 because you forgot to think about nutrition before your long run. As we say in my house, not an option. Rule number one: Begin fueling before fatigue sets in. Depending on the intensity and length of your run, you can start as early as 40 minutes, but definitely send your muscles some sugar before 60 minutes. Take in carbs in small doses—a half or full gel, two or three Clif Shot Bloks, several Starbursts, or a dried fig or two—every 30 to 45 minutes from there on out. Be sure to take a few sips of water or a sports drink along with whatever you eat. It speeds digestion and allows your system to absorb the carbs better. (A word about sports drinks: They're not water, so be sure to test before a race. They've been known to irritate sensitive gastrointestinal tracts. If you use them, be sure to factor their calories into your nutrition plans.)

Rule number two: Training runs are the time to practice what timing, flavors, and fuel sources work for you. Ideally, run on terrain similar to what you'll be racing on. Try eating two Espresso Love GUs on your 12-miler and see if you're about to retch or could suck down another.

Rule number three: On a long run, drink when you're thirsty. Despite some significant media hype about overhydrating, the most rational advice is to drink when your body tells you to. Another equally reasonable way to think about hydration is to replace what you sweat out. But knowing you soak through a sports bra doesn't answer the question of how much you've lost. Instead, weigh yourself naked before and after a typical run. Let's say you weigh 133 before you head out the door, and 90 minutes later, you are down to 131. Then, next time, you know you need to try to quaff about 32 ounces (16 ounces = 1 pound) on the road.

Run LIKE THIS MOTHER
PLOP, PLOP, FIZZ, DRINK

It might be sacrilegious to admit here, but I don't like Gatorade. Maybe if I was running across Death Valley in August, I'd chug-a-lug a bottle of the antifreeze-colored sports drink, but otherwise it seems too heavy and salty to me. Yet I sweat more than a pimply teenage boy before prom, so I need to drink something to replace the fluid and electrolytes that stream out of every. single. pore on my face and body.

Which led me to Nuun, electrolyte tablets that fizz like Alka-Seltzer when dropped into a bottle of water. Wait 2 minutes and—*voilà!*—you have a sugar-free sports drink that is effervescent instead of dense, and a pleasure to sip, instead of a pain to choke down. Think mild flavors like tri-berry, caffeinated Kona cola (Dimity's favorite), and orange ginger (my fave). These 7-calorie tablets replenish electrolytes like sodium and potassium, not carbohydrates, which is ideal for me because I like to eat my calories, not drink them.

Still not convinced? It works very well as a sugar-free ginger ale alternative when the kiddos are sick.

WHAT TO EAT AND DRINK AFTER

Your run may be done, but—get ready for a tough assignment—you have to keep eating. (You're excused from this taxing work if you've run less than 60 minutes. If it's mealtime, have at it. Otherwise, you can just go about your busy life without noshing.) Your body needs certain nutrients to build muscle tissue and make fitness gains after your workout. Carbs, in particular, are important because they help restock your glycogen (again, fancy-speak for energy) stores; protein helps repair muscle damage.

Any time you run longer than an hour, focus on refueling—and fast. There's a 20-minute window after exercise when the body is very receptive to getting glycogen back into the muscles. Alas, that is also the same time frame when your young kids are clamoring for attention because they missed momma during your 14-mile run. Keep your priorities in order as best you can.

To determine how many carbs you need within that hectic window, divide your body weight in half. If you weigh 140 pounds, you need 70 grams (or 280 calories) of simple carbohydrates. Also, aim to take in some protein during those first 20 post-run minutes to kick-start the healing of microscopic tears in your muscles. Dimity and I both like a tall glass of low-fat chocolate milk (16 ounces = 316 calories, 52 grams of carbs, 16 grams of protein) because it hits both bases: sugar and protein. Other quick-grab options: an English muffin with peanut butter or a yogurt and banana.

Within an hour of that snack, get ready to eat more! This time, put together a full meal with both carbohydrates and protein, ideally in a 4:1 carb-to-protein ratio. Athletes should aim to gobble up 10 to 20 grams of protein within an hour of finishing a workout. The protein helps repair muscle damage, and according to a 2006 study published in the journal *Medicine and Science in Sports and Exercise,* eating both carbs and protein together actually increases your muscle glycogen levels more than eating carbohydrates alone. A bean burrito, some minestrone with crusty whole-grain bread, or pasta with meat sauce does your body good.

Even though the Herculean effort you put out during a run feels like it entitles you to eat with abandon—a row of Oreos, anyone?—during the rest of the day, don't be deceived. Certainly it's fine to get yourself a cone when you treat the kids to gelato or to snack mid-afternoon on a small bag of salt and vinegar chips. Running is an effective counterbalance to such indulgences, but it doesn't get you off the hook. Not to sound like a food pyramid, but smart choices throughout the day, including a variety of carbs, protein, fiber, fruits, and veggies, give you get-up-and-go for all your runs—and let you still crank out a report for your boss or finish sewing the daisy costume for your daughter's recital. And remember to drink throughout the day, not just before, during, and immediately after a run.

I tossed the V-8, low-fat cheese, and pureed cauliflower long ago and restocked my fridge and cupboards with my favorites. My go-to foods include yogurt, tomato soup, whole-grain bread, chèvre, hummus, pre-cooked lentils, and fruit. And, of course, bag upon bag upon bag of 99-cent penne pasta.

.2 MARATHON FOODS THAT GO THE DISTANCE
By Dimity

I short-order food for my kids—usually something in the little-known sixth food group, melted cheese—way more often than I care to admit. I'm so efficient at filling snack baggies daily with Goldfish, animal crackers, or grapes that I could easily have a second career on a factory assembly line. As I feed my kids, I lose any inspiration to cook for myself. Unfortunately, you can't train for a marathon on leftover nuggets, no matter how much you try to convince yourself ketchup qualifies as a veggie. So here's how I fueled up for mine:

♀ Smoked turkey slices rolled in deli-cut Swiss cheese: no bread or mustard—or cleanup—necessary.

♀ Pumpkin bread with chocolate chips. My Rachael Ray tip: Using mini-chocolate chips spreads out the chocolate more evenly. (I know the baking sounds daunting, but a simple recipe takes 10 minutes max to mix up. Another RR tip: Double the recipe and freeze one loaf.)

♀ Cottage cheese, rich in protein, scooped up with blue-corn tortilla chips or pretzels. Sounds gross, tastes good.

♀ Peanut M&M's: There's nutrition in them nuts, right? Maybe not, but I redeem myself by buying the snack packs, so I don't gobble them by the handful. Instead, I just eat, oh, three snack packs at a time.

♀ Peanut butter and honey on a multigrain tortilla. Yes, I eventually have to wash the knife, but pulling out one tortilla feels like less work than two slices of bread.

♀ Spinach salad with yellow peppers, broccoli, carrots, and blue cheese crumbles: Pour out the bag of pre-washed spinach, add the bag of pre-sliced broccoli and carrots and the crumbles. I do go the extra mile and cut up the pepper.

♀ Chocolate milk: Since a 2004 study found this elixir to be basically as efficient as Gatorade for recovery after exhausting exercise (which, for me, is basically every run), I'm a convert. (And Sarah is devoted to Carnation Instant Breakfast after her long runs.)

♀ Hard-boiled eggs: What could be better than Ma Nature's original recipe that is stored in its own case? And not one pot to clean up—after all, it only held boiling water—instead of the caked-on, impenetrable residue left by scrambled eggs.

♀ Bananas with peanut butter: Slather PB on the tip, take a bite. Slather, bite, slather, bite, repeat.

♀ Quesadilla with pinto beans and salsa: I cook this easy dinner only when the pan is easily available. Which is to say, it's been sitting on the stove since yesterday's lunch, with melted-on remnants of the kids' grilled cheese sandwiches still in it.

16

RACES: JUMPING IN

By Sarah

In my mid-20s, I entered a lot of races without training—scenic 10Ks, after-work 5Ks, even a half-marathon—egged on by my pals. I worked at a magazine called *City Sports*, and I was surrounded by fun-loving, competitive jocks. Although I'd run to stay in shape for about 4 years, I was just dipping my Saucony-shod toes into the real running world. One of my favorite races was a 5K corporate challenge a bunch of us desk jockeys did in San Francisco's financial district and along the Embarcadero. It still thrills me to remember our editor-in-chief, Sue, admitting she'd been motivated to run extra-fast because she was secretly worried I'd pass her. Even if I could have, I wouldn't have; I wanted to keep my slave-wages job. To think that a real athlete—Sue's ultimate Frisbee team were national champions the following year—felt threatened by me boosted my sports ego. (Which was puny back then, Dimity. Really.)

My racing confidence was bolstered again by running the San Francisco Half Marathon with my good pal Dorothy. She was hardcore, always running before work despite having to be at her financial job desk at 5:30 A.M. She got up so early it's more accurate to say she was doing late-night runs instead of early morning ones. Yet somehow I started inching ahead of her around mile 5, and by mile 8 Dorothy told me to go on ahead of her. Alone, I focused on my surroundings. I'd never been around so many runners, and my memories of the race are a blur of yellow, red, blue, and green T-shirts being buffeted by a stiff ocean breeze as we all cruised up San Francisco's Great Highway. I also remember craving Coke, randomly. The typical coastal fog was nowhere in sight, and my mood was as festive as the scene.

A few months later, I joined a master's swimming team because, at the age of 24, I had finally taught myself how to put my face in the water and alternate breath (on both the right and left sides). I was excited to make up for lost time as a genuine swimmer, so I hit the pool more than the pavement. I was woefully slow, barely out-touching Vic, a grandfather who had had triple bypass surgery.

PRACTICAL *Motherly* ADVICE
GETTING TO THE STARTING LINE

Never toed the line? Sorry, no excuse. You owe it to yourself to try a race at least once. Some ways to talk (or trick) yourself into pinning on a number:

♀ Consider your goal. Looking to lose weight? Train for at least a 10K so you'll be forced to put in some longer, calorie-spewing miles. Want to get faster? Challenge yourself with a 5K and commit to dragging your butt to the track. Looking to just finish? Again, a 5K is a smart choice.

♀ Season well. A 5K at the stroke of midnight on January 1 sounds like a great way to ring in the New Year, but training in the dark and cold of November and December may pop your cork. Long runs in preparation for a spring marathon pose the same pitfalls, although it also means your 26.2 is behind you before summer heat and humidity arrive. Choose a race that lets you train in friendly weather, and you're more likely to stay committed to your goal.

♀ Grab a friend. Think locally—your running partner, your neighbor, that sporty mom at preschool—or choose faraway friends with whom you can text about today's mileage. We know women who have picked a destination race, convinced their high school buddies to join them, then ran among the palm trees and enjoyed post-race facials and catch-ups.

♀ Don't shortchange yourself. No quicker way to get turned off of racing than to jump into one with zero training. (Hello, torn Achilles!) Training times vary: Budget 6 weeks to prep for a 5K, 8 weeks for a 10K, 2 months or more for a half-marathon, and at least 3 months for a full 26.2.

♀ Pony up. Maybe I'm a cheapskate (although I prefer the label *thrifty*), but once I've paid for a race, I know I'll train for and run it. More incentive: hotel reservations and a plane ticket. It's hard to bail when you have to go through the hassle of canceling reservations and paying at least $100 change-ticket fee.

♀ Talk it up. The more people you tell, the more people you'll owe a race report to the morning after. Wanting to save face will keep you from bailing. "Uh, gee, yeah, I didn't train so I blew it off" just doesn't have the same ring to it as, "I broke an hour for a 10K!"

TAKE IT *From* A MOTHER
WHAT'S YOUR MOST MEMORABLE RACE?

"Race for the Cure. I run it with my sister-in-law, a two-time survivor of breast cancer, every year. It is her race. She will always beat me, and that's the way it should be."

—PAMELA (top three reasons for running: "I love it, I love it, I love it.")

"The Vancouver, B.C., marathon stands out because it was my first time breaking 4 hours. I overheard a woman saying it was her 100th marathon and she wanted to run it in under 4 hours, so I figured she was pretty experienced in pacing and followed her, unbeknownst to her. Afterwards, I thanked her, and she was so gracious. A real inspiration."

—SHERYL (likes the treadmill best when she's pregnant. "It's close to a bathroom.")

"Race for the Mountains in Breckenridge, Colorado. It's a trail race I created to combine my love of running and the mountains with my passion for educational projects for children in Pakistan and Afghanistan."

—SHANNON (started mountain2mountain.com, an educational charity.)

"The Kelly Butte Classic, an 8K in Eugene, Oregon. I ran it when I was on vacation, and the weather was wonderful; it was a breeze to run after training in Texas humidity. I placed second in my age group, which made me so proud, since Eugene is the running capital of the nation."

—SHELLEY (in love with trails near San Antonio. "I know their curves, and I can always conquer them.")

"The Peachtree Road Race in Atlanta. When I moved there, my brother said the reason you live in Atlanta is to run the Peachtree. I entered, along with 50,000 other runners, and made it an annual event."

—AMY (dream place to run: Paris. "Everything is bliss in Paris.")

"Prickly Pear 10-mile trail run in San Antonio: the food, the people, the relaxed atmosphere."

—KAT (replenishes after a run with coffee. "I know, I know. But caffeine is a food group to me.")

"The Yiasou Greek Fest 5K in Charlotte, North Carolina. In 2001, I finally broke 20 minutes, which I had trained my butt off for (literally). I didn't win an award because of the stellar field, but it was that field that pushed me to run my best."

—CHRISTINE (dream running date: Paula Radcliffe.)

"The Bix 7 in Davenport, Iowa, which is close to my hometown. Competing in this race every summer turned into a way to return home and have a bit of a family reunion. It became a tradition, and my twin sister and I have inspired many friends and family members to run it with us over the years. It's a challenging course in brutal heat and humidity, but the crowd support during and the revelry after the race are unparalleled."

—TAMARA (best part of a run: "finishing it, and knowing I've done something good for myself.")

Yet everyone on the team was required to compete in meets, so I pulled on my Speedo and goggles instead of shorts and sunglasses. Even though I was also smitten with mountain biking, I was too intimidated to jump into triathlons. Except for two marathons in the late 1990s, I didn't do road races again until the next millennium.

After having the kiddos, I debated trying to recapture the excitement of my youthful races, but money was tighter. I couldn't justify coughing up 40 clams for some bananas, a cup or two of Gatorade, and a tee splattered with sponsor logos to run a distance I normally do anyway. I signed up for a handful of half-marathons and another marathon, but for 5Ks and 10Ks, it seemed like too much money, not enough miles.

The Cinco de Mayo 10K here in Portland put the racing bug back in my wicking baseball cap. I'd been training a few weeks for the Nike Marathon, and my coach wanted to see what I was capable of. A friend's hubby, Dave, was running it as well, so I had company at the start, which is a race pre-req for me. Truth be told, another reason I'd shied away from races is I get timid and nervous at the start if I don't have a buddy or two by my side. And, in case you haven't noticed by now, my competitive fires run hot, so I thrive on having someone to challenge.

I didn't know much about the race going into it, which was a good thing or I might not have gotten out of bed that morning. (Another reason I hadn't donned a race number in a while is that pre-race dread I feel as I lie sleepless in bed before the alarm goes off. I resign myself to the fact that I brought this on myself, so I have to suck it up, get up, and deal.) For about 2 miles, the 10K climbs up one of Portland's longest hills. But proving ignorance is bliss, I showed up raring to go. I must have eaten my Wheaties that morning because the endless hill that always loomed large in my imagination was less steep than I'd always thought. I was able to bound up the hill, passing runners the entire climb.

As I loped along, I thought back to my first-ever 10K. I'm not certain, but I think it was called the Fleet Week 10K, but the course was unforgettable. The race was the only time of the year runners were given access to the Bay Bridge, allowing us to run over the glistening San Francisco Bay to Treasure Island, the island halfway between S.F. and Oakland where the 1939 World's Fair was held. Living in the City by the Bay, it's impossible to not be transfixed by the area's natural beauty and rich history, and this race captured both. The exhilaration of running on a normally cars-only bridge, with a sweeping view of the East Bay hills, canceled out any reservations I had about not being trained or any nerves about being surrounded by "real" runners. Plus, my man, John, ran the race with me all 3 years I did it. We were always as eager as two ponies before the start of that race, which, alas, was canceled in the early 1990s.

Back in Portland, at the halfway point of the Cinco de Mayo 10K, I realized it was literally all downhill from here, so I opened it up and let gravity have its way with all 162 pounds of me. I spied Dave's shaggy head a mere 200 meters ahead of me. I couldn't catch him, so I picked out a woman in a bright green U of O tee to catch up to, and maybe even pass. With almost every step, I was closing the gap with her. If I was floating on the way up, I was flying on the way down. I realized I never feel this elated during a solo run.

That, in a nutshell, is why I'm once again game to enter races. They bring out a whole new dimension to your running. Sure, you can push yourself during a tempo run or intervals, but nothing compares with suffering more than you thought you could, having a crowd cheer you on while you do, being completely drained as you cross the line, and yet feeling euphoric the whole time. Jill, a mom of three, puts it perfectly when she says she feels "exhausted, and so completely energized after a race."

In Portland that spring day, I felt jubilant when I crossed the line in 51:38, with an average pace of 8:19, a 10K best for me at the time. I was *en fuego!* Later, perusing the results online, I was surprised to find out I placed tenth among the master's women. Yee-ha! Back in San Francisco, I don't think I ever broke an hour for 6.2 miles, but at that time, believe it or not, going fast wasn't the point. In my novice racing days, it was about bolstering my confidence and building my identity as a runner. Those races, drenched in my mind in California sunshine, were my initiation into a tribe of racers among whom I now feel at home.

Forget what I wrote about entry fees: To me, that membership is priceless.

TAKE IT *From* A MOTHER
WHAT'S YOUR IDEAL RACING DISTANCE?

"10K, because it's longer than I have time to run on a daily basis, but it's short enough that I don't need to fit in a lot of training."

—TILNEY (worst 5K: "First mile in under 7:30, and I'm not a 7:30 runner. I thought I was going to die at mile 2.5.")

"15K or higher. It's just not worth the hassle of getting to the race and making sure the family is taken care of for anything less. Plus, it's tough to pay the entry fee for anything shorter than a race that doesn't push me at least a little."

—MEGAN (qualified for Boston the morning her period began. "I channeled all that super PMS energy into the race.")

"10-milers and half-marathons because they are long enough to fully deserve a reward, and you really need to train for them."

—CHRISTINE (dream running date: too X-rated to share.)

"13.1 because it's just enough distance to give you a wonderful hurt."

—JILL (hates to admit that weight training, which she loathes, has made her a stronger runner.)

"Half-marathon because the training doesn't invade my life. I feel very strong at that distance, and it doesn't wreak havoc on my body—I can actually walk the next day."

—JULIE (mantra, adopted from yoga instructor: Give thanks to obstacles in life because they help us grow.)

"The marathon. I love the feeling of accomplishment I get from finishing. I love being able to run for a long time and a long way."

—WENDY (has run more than fifty marathons.)

"Doesn't matter. I love every distance. As long as I have a bib on and a race to run, I'll be there."

—TINA (doesn't drink soda because "it makes my restless leg syndrome act up, which leads to insomnia, which leads to tired and cranky Tina who does not want to run.")

Run LIKE THESE MOTHERS
PICKING THE RIGHT DISTANCE

Waffling between a 5K and a 50K? (OK, a 5K and a 10K?) Here's our totally biased view of the pros and cons of the most popular race distances.

5K (3.1 MILES)
Love It Because:

♀ Can crank one out, shower, and still be early to brunch (or happy hour).

♀ Lets you shift into fifth gear and stay there the entire distance.

♀ Chance to run with kiddies. They're content to be in a jogging stroller for that distance or can run it solo once they hit about second grade.

♀ Lots of opportunities to support charitable causes by simply hitting the pavement.

Hate It Because:

♀ Can be crowded, especially the first mile, so it's hard to get a rhythm as you bob and weave through the throngs of people.

♀ So short! Unless you run super-speedy, it almost feels like you still need to do another workout. (That's Sarah's take. Dimity is beyond cool with 3.1 miles in a day, no matter what pace.)

♀ Setting a PR for veteran runners probably takes lots of laps around the track, which means more time and forethought for a workout.

♀ Sometimes the race fee feels steep for a half-hour run.

10K (6.2 MILES)
Love It Because:

♀ Distance is long enough to test endurance but short enough to keep the hammer down the whole way (hey, it is a race!).

♀ Feels like a workout without turning you into a noodle for the rest of the day.

♀ Training takes focus but doesn't monopolize your life.

Hate It Because:

⟋ Getting harder to find ones that aren't mob scenes.

⟋ It doesn't offer as much challenge as other distances. On 5Ks, you can work speed and leave it all out there because 3.1 miles isn't crazy long. Meanwhile, half-marathons and fulls are major tests of endurance. A 10K? Neither here nor there.

⟋ It's easy to go out too hard, leaving you sputtering halfway through the race.

HALF-MARATHON

Love It Because:

⟋ Requires determined but not over-the-top training.

⟋ A valid excuse to visit Napa Valley, Disney World, or some other vacation destination. (Run first, then chill.)

⟋ Crossing the finish line feels like major accomplishment.

⟋ Bragging rights: Just using the words "I finished" and "marathon" in a sentence—regardless what other words are in it—makes you feel like a rock star.

⟋ Often combined with marathons. When you see the half-marathon turn off and know that other runners/suckers are only halfway and you're nearly done, the feeling of relief is sweet!

Hate It Because:

⟋ On bad race days, the wheels fall off around mile 10, and you've still got about 25 percent of the race left.

⟋ Stop to pee at porta-potty or just hold it?

⟋ Have to figure out a nutrition and hydration system that works for you, or you'll be faced with multiple visits to the honey bucket.

⟋ Long training runs eat into weekend time, requiring arrangements with the spouse.

continued on page 134

MARATHON

Love It Because:

9 Makes you dig into emotional and physical reserves you don't usually mine.

9 Lets you cross off an item on your life to-do list.

9 Makes you feel almost as proud as the day your babies were born.

9 Nearly guilt-free consumption of Mint Milanos and chocolate ice cream after a long run.

9 Taper makes you feel like Kate Winslet on the bow of the *Titanic*: invincible.

Hate It Because:

9 Makes you dig into emotional and physical reserves you don't usually mine.

9 Long training runs sap your energy and patience for the rest of the day.

9 An open invitation to overuse injuries.

9 Training—and the can-you-watch-the-kids negotiations so you can do the long runs—takes on life of its own.

9 Mile 22 makes you feel like Kate Winslet after the iceberg: sunk.

.2 PRE-RACE BEAUTY DOS AND DON'TS
By Sarah

The exertion of a 15-mile training run or 10K race is taxing enough without adding in personal hygiene screw-ups. My misery is your gain. Lessons I've learned from the ground up:

- Don't get a pedicure the week before a race. It's a waste of money because your Cha-Ching Cherry tootsies will look hammered at the end.

- Also, don't go crazy clipping your toenails beforehand. If you leave a sharp corner, it can dig into its neighboring toe with every step. Cut your toenails straight across.

- But don't take foot matters into your own hands. I made that rookie mistake before my first marathon, hacking away at my cheese-rind calluses the night before the race. Before I realized it, I'd left my tender feet overexposed, inviting blisters.

- Rub self-tanner on your gams so they look as sleek as they are strong. Finish-line photos highlight dimples and puckers I swear aren't there in everyday life. When my skin is an even bronze tone, I look like a thoroughbred, not a mare put out to pasture.

- Don't forget to shave, pits included. Do it a day or two before the race; the night before or morning of, you might be too nervous and draw blood. Plus, the raw skin in your pits, not used to being exposed to miles of sweat, could get irritated.

- Don't wax or pluck your brows too drastically. It isn't until sweat is streaming unimpeded from your forehead into your eyes that you realize why we have bushy eyebrows.

- At the risk of sounding like your mother, don't forget sweat-proof sunscreen. And test the sweat-proof claim before race day: You know that your quads will scream, but stinging eyes is just too much pain.

- Don't debut a short new haircut if you're wearing a running hat. You might be mistaken for your 13-year-old half-brother in a race photo.

17

THE MARATHON: **THE MOTHER OF ALL RACES**

By Sarah

The younger you are, the more firsts you rack up: first gas-induced smile, first true smile, first haircut, first real food, first poop in the tub, first repetition of a swear word said by exasperated parent. As you get older, the firsts dwindle with age. At 5, you still have lots of proverbial cherries to pop: starting kindergarten, losing a tooth, riding two wheels, until you get to the stale point where the only first left is the popping of another kind of cherry.

Running, though, gives you an opportunity to crack open the spine of a spankin' new journal, devoted solely to your next round of firsts. And there's nothing more deserving of a page or 2—or 20—than your first marathon. Like surviving labor, crossing the finish line of a 26.2-mile race is a testament to perseverance, discipline, dedication, and a few other multisyllabic words often found on inspirational posters hanging on office walls. The race is a huge accomplishment, of course, but it's really the months of training that change your life and perspective. During the no-glory, no-spectators training miles, you discover how hard you can push yourself, how persistent you need to be, and how to call forth motivation when you'd rather just call for a pizza.

There are as many reasons to challenge yourself to train for and conquer a marathon as there are steps taken in one (76,000, for all you math geeks, Dimity included). A partial list of what spurs someone to take on 26 miles, 385 yards: a desire to see how tough you are. The wish to show your kids they can do anything once they set their minds to it. The wish to show *yourself* you can do anything once you set your mind to it. An excuse to get out of the house. The chance to shorten your bucket list. A way to lose weight, to raise money for a cause. A reason to justify spending endless hours gossiping with a girlfriend. A dare. A lark. Insert your own here:

_____.

My first was the San Francisco Marathon in 1998. My reasons for doing it were mostly linked to a short-term move from the City by the Bay to Chicago to be with my then-boyfriend, Jack. I thought it would be fun to feel a tie to my beloved San Francisco while I was living in an unfamiliar city and then have a definite reason—marathon weekend—to go back there. I also wanted a goal that would help pass those lonely hours when friends were a long-distance call, not a bike ride, away. Plus, I wanted the bragging rights that come with going the distance. A part of me felt I would become a real runner once I finished a marathon.

I had several friends who had run one, including a former co-worker named Julie. She'd run the San Francisco Marathon in 1991, and I'd cheered her on near mile 26. I watched with such awe as runners of all shapes and sizes trotted toward the finish line. Some wore scowls, but the majority had smiles worthy of a Colgate toothpaste commercial. After the race, it seemed Julie was buzzing on the ultimate runner's high. I wanted a swig of that elixir.

I didn't follow any set training plan. (I cringe now, admitting that.) Instead I honed my English-major math skills by increasing my mileage by about 10 percent each week. A 10-mile long run one Sunday lengthened to an 11-mile one the next week. I figured running three, maybe four times a week would get me through. However, I knew I had to do at least one 20-mile training run.

After doing all my weekday runs along Chicago's lakefront—I'm convinced I wore a groove in the concrete of Oak Street Beach—I craved new vistas for my first venture into 20-mile territory. So one muggy Sunday, I headed out of the city to a rail-to-trail conversion. I started running with no clue where I was headed, only hoping the paved trail stretched 10 miles in front of me.

I had one water bottle, a few bucks, and a wild berry PowerBar with me. By about mile 8, I was sopping wet with sweat. Despite a leafy canopy, I was wilting. I rationed my water, but I drained the last drops by about mile 14. I had an hour or more left without any hydration. I felt desperation creeping up on me as my spit turned syrupy and my legs got heavy. Then I spotted it: a 7-Eleven, an oasis. I stumbled toward it like a shipwreck survivor. The bell tinkled as I opened the door, and a welcome blast of A/C hit me.

It's not in the Guinness Book, but I firmly believe I set a world record for chugging a Gatorade in that convenience store. Then I refilled the bottle with water from the pop dispenser before resuming my shuffle. I collapsed into Jack's Jetta after about three and a half hours, making a giant wet spot on the scratchy upholstery seats. Everything hurt; even my right forearm felt crampy after clutching a bottle for so many miles. I was quaking in my Adidases at the thought of running an additional 10K on top of the distance I'd just covered.

Run LIKE THIS MOTHER
NO REST FOR THE WEARY

The night before a marathon, don't expect to sleep well, if at all. Expect to toss, turn, and fret. Every marathoner has been there, but I deserve special commendation for braving an especially heinous night before a race. It was 2003, and Jack, Phoebe, and I were in Calistoga, California, so I could run my third marathon: the Napa Valley. We had never gone on a weekend getaway as a family; it was my present to myself for turning 37. We were staying in a small B&B that, fortunately, only housed us and the innkeeper.

Phoebe was 14 months old, and I had weaned her days before. We'd both savored a final breastfeeding session on Tuesday morning. This was Saturday night. I must have been psychic, sensing what was coming, as I went to bed at 8 P.M., even earlier than usual, and fell asleep shockingly fast. At midnight, though, my sweet slumber was broken by Phoebe crying in her Pack 'n' Play. Even though she'd been a sound sleeper since she was about 8 weeks old—don't hate me!—something was bothering that child that night. Maybe it was being weaned or sleeping in a strange bed, but she was clearly not happy.

Phoebe continued to cry inconsolably for nearly 4 hours. Yes, 4 hours. (The time I was, once again, trying to break on the race course the next day.) Crying, wailing, thrashing, quivering. "You've *got* to stop crying," I begged, pleaded, and even threatened a few times. "Momma's got a big race in a few hours!" Nothing calmed her down. Countless times I considered whipping out a milk-filled boob, but I was resolute: She was weaned. Call me heartless, but I was done nursing. Meanwhile, Jack slept like a, uh, baby the entire time. I hated him for that, but didn't want to wake him up because I knew I'd need him to take care of Phoebe and me, post-race, the next day.

Finally, in desperation, I put her in bed between Jack and me because I had to get off my feet. (I know, I know: Why hadn't I tried that simple tactic before?) At long last, Phoebe calmed down and started to doze off. Every so often, though, she'd be racked by one of those post-crying-jag shudders, sending a tremor across the entire mattress and jarring me out of the butterfly-light sleep into which I'd fallen.

It was futile. I got up, donned my racing garb, ate a banana and an energy bar, and walked the mile and a half to the start line. I ended up running my fastest marathon to date (4:01:02), but for months afterward, I wondered if I could have broken 4:00 if I'd only gotten a few more hours of shut-eye.

The next year, though, I was pleased to read a study reported in the September 2004 *Journal of Sports Medicine and Physical Fitness*. Researchers found it's the sleep you get *two* nights before a competition that really matters, not the night before. Among the 22 study participants, VO_2 peak, or how efficiently your body can process oxygen, was not adversely affected after one night of sleep deprivation; it was lowest two days after sleep deprivation.

So I can't really blame Phoebe. Still, I can put a mental asterisk next to that finishing time—and maybe even hold it over her head when she becomes a sulky, ungrateful teenager.

Ever the optimist, I still set my sights on breaking 4 hours in that July marathon, despite never setting foot on a track during my 4 months of training or even cranking up the intensity of my runs. I won't take you step-by-*ouch*-step through the race, but here are my standout memories: Running the first mile across the magical Golden Gate Bridge in a light fog, feeling ebullient. Joy turning to desolation as I chugged for miles in the then-dilapidated China Basin and Third Street area, where the only sign of life along the race course was still-slumbering homeless people. Bursting out with laughter at one woman's T-shirt that read, "I want to be Martha. That bitch can do anything!" Having my spirits brightened again a few miles later when rowdy Kate and Sarah greeted me near the Rose Garden in Golden Gate Park—and then me throwing up, into my cupped hands, the flat Coke I'd asked them to bring for me. Being thrilled my dear friend Stacy jumped into the race at mile 19 to run me in. And telling her at about mile 24 that breaking 4 hours was a ridiculous goal for me because my thighs had turned to cement. Crossing the line in 4:04:03 and hobbling to a spot of grass to try to lower my broken-down body to the ground.

Even though I had pictured the marathon for 4 months, I had no idea how dramatically and unexpectedly my mood would swing during it. I'd heard plenty of stories, but hearing about 26.2 and running 26.2 is like babysitting versus having a few rugrats of your own: You can't really know what a marathon is like until you go the distance yourself.

Just as distinctly I remember the conversation I had that afternoon with my good friend Bevin, who had recently run her first 26.2-miler, the St. George Marathon in southwest Utah. I was cashed out on my down-filled sofa with my legs propped up. Despite the cushy couch, I was far from comfortable. As soon as Bevin answered the phone, I blurted out, "Why didn't you tell me the marathon was going to be so hard?" She laughed and explained she didn't want to scare me off. We commiserated and kvetched. (Fast forward four years: Bevin gave birth to her first child,

Sean, 2 weeks before I had my first baby. "How brutal is childbirth?" I asked her a few days after he was born. "Be honest. Don't hold out on me like you did with the marathon.")

Bevin and I vowed to never run another one. A promise she's kept—and one I didn't. Less than 16 months later I was toeing the line at the New York City Marathon. As with childbirth, the memory of the pain had receded, and running for about 4 hours straight sounded like a grand idea. And this time it was, thanks to better training (two 20-milers) and more realistic expectations. It was actually an enjoyable experience, if you can call slamming into a wall at mile 21 "enjoyable." Since then, I've become a bit of a junkie: I've gone on to run a total of five marathons, and even before I crossed the line in the fifth, I was mulling over which one would be my sixth.

Why am I hooked? Mostly, I adore the journey to the starting line—or, in other words, I thrive on the work it takes to get to race day. The weeks and months of training stretch in front of me like the Yellow Brick Road, and I can't help but smile and click my heels. I love the purpose that accompanies the this-is-my-workout-today certainty and the accomplishment I feel nearly every day. I come alive with the ebb and flow of long runs: "I feel fantastic: I want to run forever," followed close on the heels by, "That's it: I can't go another step. I'm hitchhiking home!" I thrive on the pride of seeing my weekly mileage jump higher than ever, and I chuckle at thinking of an 8-mile run as short. Believe it or not, each time I haven't wanted the training to end.

But like all journeys, the training does come to an end, and all that's left is 26.2. Waiting for the starting gun, I tell myself, "I've done the work, and now I'm ready to show it." I set off, shored up for the flood of feelings to hit. There's euphoria at the start, when I barely feel my feet touching the pavement, then I settle into a steady groove, followed by a spirit-crushing low around mile 18 or 20, then a crescendo-like high as I approach the finish line.

At least that's the general pattern. I've had good marathons, where the crush hardly bleeped on my radar, and I've had one where I felt disconsolate nearly the entire race. I returned to San Fran for the Nike Marathon 9 years later, still striving to break 4:00. Once again I didn't meet my goal—three kids under age 6 might have had something to do with that—and I emotionally crumpled at the finish line. If only my legs could have moved as fast during the race as my tears flowed after it. Within hours after crossing the line, however, I was proud of my effort in that 26.2-miler. Although it was my fourth time covering that daunting distance, I came to realize that it's impossible to not feel special on marathon day, no matter how many times you've run one or how the race goes.

Yet I was still bound and (fiercely) determined to run a marathon in less than 4 hours. I knew from past experience I needed two things: a flat course and a coach. I chose the Eugene Marathon,

TAKE IT *From* A MOTHER
HAVE YOU EVER USED A PACE GROUP IN A MARATHON TO HELP YOU REACH YOUR GOAL TIME?

"Yes, it's one less thing to think about. All you have to do is follow the flag; even I can handle that!"

—JUNKO (top three reasons why she runs: sanity, health, and because she has to. "It's the one thing in my life purely for me.")

"I started my first marathon with the 3:40 pace group because I hoped to qualify for Boston. I loved the idea of having someone to help me keep pace. I had a female pacer with a beautiful spirit. Unfortunately, my body gave out at mile 11.5, and I could no longer keep up. Those miles that I ran with that group were my more cherished memories from the marathon. I plan to use a more realistic pace group in future races."

—MELANIE (3-year-old's description of her after a wind-blown run: "You look crazy.")

"I have started with pacing groups, but I have always ditched them at some point because I felt the need to run my own race. I try not to get too technical with my running; I don't own a Garmin and don't calculate my workouts to the exact pace detail. It takes the fun out of running for me."

—SHERI (longest distance she's run: 26.2 miles, with a 6-mile walk afterward to find a taxi in New York City.)

"I haven't used them because it's more comfortable for me to run some early miles slower and then later ones faster. But that hasn't worked out for me in terms of helping me meet my goal. In my next marathon, after I give birth to my second baby, I think I might try to run with a slower pace group to start, then finish the race on my own."

—CHRISTINE (has run five marathons. "But only one good one: San Jose.")

"Yes, to come in under 4 hours in the Phoenix marathon, we made sure to keep ahead of the 9:00 pace group as long as possible."

—SARA (first post-partum run was at 2 weeks. "I was going crazy watching people run the trail next to our house.")

an easy 2-hour drive south of Portland, because it was building a reputation as a fast, PR-friendly course. And I was fortunate enough to enlist Lynn Jennings as my coach. The pieces were in place, and I just needed to stay true to the tasks Lynn set out for me. The beauty of the workouts she gave me were that they were hard enough to be challenging but still within my grasp. (My fave? The one I later dubbed The. Best. Workout. Ever., which consisted of 4 × 1,200 at the track, then 5 tempo miles on the road, then back to the track for 2 × 1 mile). Lynn's workouts made me push myself, yet they also allowed me to succeed, thus building my confidence along with my speed, fitness, and endurance. Midway through my 3-month training for Eugene, Lynn and I both knew that, barring injury or illness, I'd break 4 hours. It just became a question of by how much.

The answer ended up being nearly seven and a half minutes—more than eight minutes off my previous personal best. Even now, months later, I tear up remembering it.

Now the question is, can I beat that? I can certainly try. My running buddies Jill and Mary like to call a marathon "the 26.2-mile victory lap," celebrating all the hard work and effort a runner puts out in the months leading up to the race. I plan on taking a couple more laps in this lifetime.

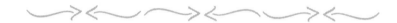

.2 SAY CHEESE: HOW TO GET THE PERFECT RACE PIC
By Dimity

If you're like me, you have tons of pictures of your kids, your kids with their dad, your kids with their grandparents, your kids with their friends, your kids with the dog. Yet because I'm typically the one behind the shutter, I have very few shots of myself. Which is fine most of the time—the dark circles under my eyes don't need to be saved for posterity, thanks—but I do want proof I ran a race. And ran it well.

I love receiving the post-race e-mail with images of me. Then I scrutinize the shots, and I realize I'm sporting a grimace, exposing a fat roll, or—the worst—looking like I'm walking when I'm not. I don't have many time goals like Sarah, but I do have a race-related goal: a picture I'd actually order. So I called the experts at Brightroom, the photographers in those ubiquitous blue vests who shoot races nationwide, and got these tips for a Kodak moment:

♀ Although race photogs try to shoot every runner, people who stand out tend to catch their eyes as they shoot a sea of runners. Easy ways to be noticed: Wear a bright top, make eye contact with the photographer, smile, and if you're up for it, give a thumb's up or wave (no middle fingers, please). If you're running with a pal, put your arm around her or grab her hand as you go by.

♀ Run on the side of the road on which the photographer is located. Don't go down the middle, unless she's on a lift in the middle of the street.

♀ Pin your number in a clear spot in the center of the top you'll be wearing for most of the race, not on your backside or on a layer you'll shed.

♀ To look your speediest, Chris Miller at Brightroom suggests thinking about running like a Kenyan for 20 yards. "Imagine you're floating, so your feet spend as little time on the ground as possible," he says.

♀ Don't wear the race T-shirt. The more fitted your outfit, the sleeker you'll look. "A parachute of a cotton tee billowing in the wind never makes anybody look good," Miller says.

♀ Do wear a skirt, which eradicates the unsightly crotch bulge shorts create after, oh, about ten steps. If you're not a skirt fan, tight compression shorts or capris are other options.

♀ Don't tailgate. For a clean, solo shot, give yourself some space between you and the runners around you.

♀ Baseball hats cast shadows over your face, especially at the finish line, where photogs tend to shoot from above. If you wear one, take it off and raise it in the air, turn it around, or, at the very least, tilt it up.

♀ Speaking of finish lines, do not look down at your watch to hit the stop button as you cross it. "That's our biggest problem," admits Miller. "Adding a couple seconds to your finishing time, which is probably being chip timed anyway, is worth a great shot."

18

PREGNANCY: **BABY ON BOARD**

By Sarah

I had numerous goals during my first pregnancy. Eat a healthful, varied diet. Drink plenty of water. Not fret about my daily, sometimes hourly weight gain. Forgo my daily Diet Coke. Find a doctor who wouldn't gasp when I told her I wanted to run through pregnancy. And not trip while trail running.

Seriously. I was worried a lot about catching my foot on rock or root and falling flat on my stomach. My rah-rah doc would have told me the baby was well insulated in amniotic fluid for the first two trimesters at least, but still I obsessed about staying upright from the get-go. During my road runs, I was carefree, but on my weekly trail runs, I was as high stepping as a Tennessee walking horse.

Even so, I did my best to enjoy every stride I took during my pregnancy. I loved the idea of running while pregnant. Before I ever got knocked up, I'd marvel when I'd see a pregnant woman running. I'd stare at her belly and think it must bounce up and down like breasts in a bargain-basement sports bra. How annoying and uncomfortable! But when it was my turn to run with a bun in the oven, I was pleased to find my bulging belly was hard and stayed firmly in place as I bounded along.

My pregnancy running routine was to do an hour-long trail run every Saturday. I treasured that time in the woods, communing with nature and my baby. In the hustle-bustle of my everyday life—registering at Babies R Us, researching cloth versus disposable diapers, and tackling extra writing assignments so I could take 6 weeks off post-baby—I didn't pause much to contemplate the life growing within me. But on my runs, I turned inward and talked downward. I treated my unborn child like a running partner, calling the baby's attention to an interesting bird call or an especially vivid autumn leaf. I'd tell it (we didn't find out the gender beforehand) how I was feeling,

PRACTICAL *Motherly* ADVICE
RULES TO RUN BY FOR 9 MONTHS

I'm not a doctor, nor do I play one on TV, but here are some guidelines I've accumulated over the years from interviewing medical experts about exercising during pregnancy.

9 Check with your doctor to be sure you don't have any health conditions that would limit you before embarking on a prenatal exercise routine.

9 Drink plenty of water, even if you aren't thirsty; dehydration can precipitate uterine contractions.

9 Remember the acronym DUL—Drink, Urinate, and Lie down—if you feel pre-term contractions while exercising.

9 Stop exercising if you feel lightheaded or dizzy. Once something makes you feel lightheaded while pregnant, cross it off your list of activities: It's not going to get better at your next workout. (Being pregnant is not the same as having an off-day in your regular, non-preggo life.)

9 Avoid exercising on your back after your first trimester. It can compress the major vessel returning blood to your heart, lowering your blood pressure and reducing blood flow to the placenta. So ix-nay on the traditional crunches or bench presses.

9 Stop exercising and call your doctor if you have chest pains, feel contractions, or start bleeding.

mentioning that my sacroiliac joint was flaring up again or my Achilles tendon was feeling tender. Inane chatter, mainly, but occasionally I'd tell the baby about my dream of using marathon training as a way to get back in shape post-partum.

I anticipated continuing to run right up until the day I delivered. I really wanted to be one of those moms who can say, "I ran 4 miles the day I went into labor." But then, at 8 months, something fundamentally shifted. Literally, I think, and basically overnight. I don't know if my baby had descended farther into my pelvis or what, but I suddenly felt a cumbersome fullness. And my wrists and ankles started to swell every day by late afternoon, often accompanied by slight tingling in my hands. Suddenly swimming—and the osmosis effect of the water—was more appealing than pounding my body in an upright position.

TAKE IT *From* A MOTHER
DID YOU RUN DURING PREGNANCY?

"Yes, I ran through two pregnancies until the ligaments under my belly were protesting too loudly. But I was very careful with the second, since I had infertility treatments to get pregnant with her. My third pregnancy was a different story: I was unknowingly pregnant with him when I raced an Ironman. Then I sat on my butt in shock during the remainder of that pregnancy."

—KAMI (her breathing mantra: In three, out two.)

"I ran a 5K 10 days before I gave birth to my first son. I didn't put pressure on myself to perform well. I ran it in 25 minutes—amazing how well you can run without pressure! People were so surprised to see me running with my big belly, and they cheered me on. I outsprinted a guy to the finish line, which was icing on the cake!"

—JILL (not a good running buddy. "I will ditch you if you don't keep up—and I'd expect the same of you!")

"I ran up to 6 months with my first child, but no more than 3 miles. I was at the mercy of my bladder."

—CHRISTINE (strategy for dealing with period while running: Midol, Midol, Midol.)

"Yes, I told my doctor I was worried about hormonal stuff making me depressed or crazy, and she said I could do everything I had been doing: running, biking, swimming. Around the end of 6 months, though, I had some pre-term contractions, so she told me to stop and I did. I had an 8-pound baby just a few days before my due date."

—CHARITY (favorite treadmill workout: anything distracting.)

"I stopped at 15 weeks with my first because it felt strange, and after miscarrying three times while trying to have a second, I decided I'd just take it easy. The time off wasn't a problem, but the road back has been a little more difficult than I expected."

—MAGGIE (favorite running partner: her dad. "We talk about stuff that we'd never discuss otherwise.")

"No. Pregnancy is its own marathon."

—JENNIFER (motivational argument: "I had three babies with no drugs. I can gut through another mile.")

"Yes, but I had to promise my doctor I'd stick to the roads. I showed up for my first-ever appointment on crutches because that morning I had twisted my ankle badly on a trail run."

—SHANNON (worst part of running: complaining knees.)

"My doctor for my first pregnancy, back in 1996, told me not to get my heart rate above 140, which happened just walking around. So I freaked and became sedentary. The second pregnancy, the rules had changed and I ran the entire time, even the day I delivered. In an effort to consolidate information I'd been researching, I created the Web site thepregnantrunner.com. Naturally, my running slowed to more like wogging (walk/jogging) than running, but it was an accomplishment to run to the end."

—CHRISTINE (find her also at therunningcoach.com.)

As a competitive athlete, I knew how to push through discomfort and obstacles, but I realized the end weeks of pregnancy weren't like toughing out the final miles of a marathon or the last few strokes of a rowing race. My body, hard at work on finishing a job more important than any trail run, was telling me to slow down, and I listened.

Plus, I'd reached my goal: During the entire journey, I never once tripped.

Ah, what a difference 4 years and 2 fetuses make. Early on during my twin pregnancy, I got metaphorically tripped up. Seven weeks along, I went for a run. Nothing major, a 5-mile route I'd done countless times before. Yet when I got back, I was spotting. Scared and panicky, I called the doctor's office. A nurse did her best to talk me down, and I took to my bed for the day like a character out of a Victorian novel. As I lay there, one of the nurse's comments swirled in my head. "You shouldn't be running," she told me, "there's a lot at risk." It's not surprising the nurse would say this: She was talking to someone who had paid thousands of dollars undergoing in vitro fertilization to get pregnant the second time around. Plus, we weren't talking one baby but two. A more precarious pregnancy by the mere fact of its twin-ness.

As tough as it was for me, a lapsed Catholic and devoted runner, I made a classic bargain with God: Let me remain pregnant, I asked Him, and I'll give up running until after the babies are born.

When the spotting ceased within an hour or two, man, was I tempted to go back on my end of the deal. But I kept my word, and I didn't run for the duration. I quickly found keep-me-sweating, maintain-my-sanity alternatives. I rode a stationary bike, swam, used the elliptical machine, and, eventually, started pool running. (Maybe God disagrees, but despite the verbiage, I don't count this as running.)

But given the time crunch of work and already having one child, my go-to exercise during the twin pregnancy was walking. After about 5 months, I strapped on a supportive elastic belly band, carried a bottle of water, and strode around my neighborhood and even on some trails, lifting my feet high, of course. I walked until the day the twins were born. Not as impressive a statement, in my mind, as having run on their birthday, but my pride of carrying the twins full term supersedes even my sports ego.

One thing I learned during both pregnancies is how little medical professionals really know about what's OK and what's not during pregnancy. Sure, docs can say with certainty to steer clear of deli meats and blue cheese because of the risk of infection from listeria, yet they can't agree on how much exercise and exertion counts as too much.

Some doctors still tell their patients to not let their heart rate go over 140 beats per minute, despite the American College of Obstetrics and Gynecology dropping that caveat years ago. Most practitioners now suggest not getting too overheated or out of breath, both frustratingly vague recommendations. (Thus the reason I sometimes, literally, said out loud while running preggo, "Can I still carry on a conversation?" to gauge my exertion level.)

In-the-know docs say the best exercise guideline during these months is perceived exertion. While pregnant runners usually want to aim for the 5 to 8, fragmented-conversation range on the scale of 1 to 10, don't worry if an occasional hill gets you slightly more winded. Mona Shangold, M.D., director of the Center for Women's Health and Sports Gynecology in Philadelphia, once told me, "It's best for people to avoid maximal exertion during pregnancy, such as you'd give in a competitive race. But there's no evidence it's harmful." But you can still enter a race and run at a cruising pace.

One specific caveat Dr. Shangold gave was to not stop suddenly when you're doing strenuous exercise. It seems an abrupt cessation of muscle contractions can cause a rapid drop in blood pressure or blood flow—not what you want when you have someone else relying on you for oxygen and nutrients. Ease from a run to a jog to a walk, rather than just putting on the brakes at your front door or the trailhead. Build a sufficient cooldown into your routine, such as a 5-minute walk at the end of a run. Or switch to walking if your body tells you to. As Dr. Shangold told me, "It is better to err on the side of exercising too slowly rather than overdoing it."

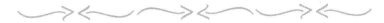

.2   RUNNING THROUGH THE CIRCLE OF LIFE
By Dimity

My grandmother died last night. I went for a run this morning. I didn't run in honor of her—a dainty woman, always in dresses, she didn't understand why anybody would run—but I ran because she, a mother of four, was gone. Really my step-grandmother, she was 93, had been struggling for months, and had a life so inimitable, it's worth a novel. So I wasn't nauseated with grief for her. She was ready for heaven. But I was sick to my stomach with the idea that mothers die, that my stepdad no longer has a mother, an anchor.

Nearly four decades into my life, I'm as naïve as I was at age 8. I'm well aware of the delicate circle of life, but certain unsavory aspects of it—kids getting cancer, women being raped, gratuitous killing of anybody—pummel me no matter how anonymous the victim is or how many times I've heard a similar story. Since I've had kids, I've added mothers who die to that list. My husband lost his mother when he was only 8, and I look at Amelia, now 6, and think, "I'd know her for just 2 more years?" I can't bear the thought.

Running doesn't cure anything, of course. But it's a temporary fix. It makes your blood flow, your lungs fill, your rhythm return. You feel in charge, like you could change something if you only set your mind to it. Like disease and tragedy, running is raw and undiscriminating, but unlike those, running leads you to believe the world spins on order, reason, and positive vibes.

As I ran this morning, I wondered whether I would be able to summon the energy to get out of bed, let alone run, when my (very healthy, lively) mom dies. Recently, when she was on yoga retreat in Mexico for a week and I couldn't dial her number for our daily, banal 5-minute check-in, I felt adrift and lonely. I can't imagine years of that feeling. She doesn't really understand why I run so much either. But without sounding too morbid—or wishing away time—I'm pretty sure I'd run the day of her funeral.

Because sometimes running is the only thing to do when you don't know what to do.

19

POST-PREGNANCY: **THE LONG ROAD BACK**

By **Dimity**

There's one in every crowd. "Oh, I ran the day before I gave birth," a Paula Radcliffe wannabe proclaims to nobody in particular, "and a week later, I was back to 6 miles, 6 days a week." I force my best social smile and say, "Good for you. Very cool." Inwardly, I'm rolling my eyes and thinking, "Hope a little sleep deprivation doesn't interfere with training for your umpteenth marathon, Ms. Overachiever."

Here's a chapter for the 99 percent of us left in her baby-powder dust. Starting to run again and finding your groove after pregnancy, like almost everything related to mothering, is much easier said than done. Six weeks post-Amelia, I remember embarking on my first run, a measly 15-minute outing, formerly known as my warmup. I slowed to a walk within 3 minutes of my "run" but willed myself through the whole 15 minutes of heavy breathing. I returned home, lacking both endorphins and hope.

There are times in your life when you need to be gentle with yourself, when being mentally tough means being stubborn enough to not beat yourself up with shouldas, wouldas, why-didn't-yas. The first 3 months post-partum, at a minimum, is one of those times. Even if you regularly got out there during pregnancy, running after the most delicate parts of your body have been stretched to unbelievable sizes (or, worse, your belly slashed) to pop out a piglet is like starting from scratch. Add in the lovely benefits accompanying new motherhood—less sleep in a week than you used to get in a night, hormones that course through your blood like Class V rapids, and generally weird feelings (this peanut belongs to me? how did that happen?)—and you're not just at ground zero, you're actually in the hole.

I have no prescription for regaining endurance, speed, or even sanity except to run when a small part of you feels twitchy enough to try it and stop when it feels like too much. Don't compare yourself to anybody, especially your former self. Don't dwell on the fact your inner thighs collide with every step. Don't hate every single bleepin' runner who blows by you. End a 25-minute run feeling strong, instead of a 45-minute one feeling defeated. And repeat this trite, annoying mantra when (not if) you feel whale-ish, turtle-ish, and unrunnerish: "It took me 9 months to get out of shape, it'll take me 9 months to get back into shape."

What I do know is that the first 9 months post-baby are equal parts elation and desperation, and running adds to the former and eases the latter. I also know most new mothers study the *What to Expect* series by Heidi Murkoff with a near biblical devotion. So here, in an all-too-familiar format, is a rough post-partum guide to the ups and downs of a running mother.

1 WEEK
What You Probably Will Be Doing

- Obsessing about pooping. What once used to be a movement you welcomed—it signaled all is clear, time to hit the road—is now cause for extreme concern. How much will it hurt? How can I even wipe?

- Crying unexpectedly. You're watching *Entertainment Tonight*, the baby has been asleep for hours, and your husband is on his way back with your favorite Indian take-out. Which is all cause for tears, of course.

- Disbelieving there are actually two of you in the house—you and your child—who need diapers. Why didn't anybody tell you you'd be wearing pads the size of diving boards?

- Going for a walk around your block. Stepping gingerly, being overly aware of any stitches, feeling completely wiped, but doing it nonetheless.

What You Will Possibly Be Doing

- Comparing your bodaciousness with that of a *Penthouse* centerfold. Your boobs are so mongo, sore, and bothersome, you'll applaud any runner with a D cup or bigger for the rest of your life.

- Pretending you're still pregnant. Even though you left the hospital with an infant in your arms, not your belly, and roughly 10 pounds of blood, placenta, and goo slithered out of your body, your bloated stomach looks like the doctor neglected to deliver the other twin.

- Fitting into your running shoes and socks. And reaching down to tie your running shoes all by yourself! What a good girl!

What You May Be Concerned About

"Every muscle in my body aches, from my shoulders to my calves.
I haven't done anything in at least 3 weeks—I spent the last weeks
of pregnancy bonding with the couch—so what's up?"

Forget races across the Sahara or Antarctic or anything else extreme: Childbirth is the hardest work-out ever, as everything from your whining neck ligaments to your kinked foot arches can attest. Whether you gave birth naturally, enhanced by an epidural, or via C-section, your body has been *worked*. Add in awkward birth positions (spread your legs as wide as a Mack truck, please), a hospital bed slightly more comfortable than a camping air mattress, and odd and new mothering actions, such as nursing, carrying a car seat/cement block, and swaying endlessly, and you've got a recipe for delayed-onset muscle soreness that lasts for weeks. If you can—a big if—sneak off for a massage with a masseuse who specializes in car-ing for pregnant women. They have a belly pillow that can accommodate your still-preggo stomach.

2 TO 4 WEEKS
What You Will Probably Be Doing

- Sitting on a couch straight up. No more plastic inflated doughnut, despite hemorrhoids with more staying power than a blackened toenail.

- Mastering the one-handed maternity bra closure, if you're breastfeeding, or if you're not, breathing a sigh of relief your Dolly P.s are slowly dwindling back to normal.

- Slithering into a sports bra and wondering if it could double as a nursing bra. Yes, it can, but make sure it's not cutting off your circulation.

- Jogging in place to see if said bra will work when it's time to hit the road. Nope, it suddenly seems as flimsy as Saran Wrap.

- Feeling a little stir crazy if you're used to regular exercise. You're daydreaming about running, especially when the baby blues hit and you need to chase them away with an endorphin rush.

What You Will Possibly Be Doing

- Getting through a trip to the grocery store without you or your babe breaking down.

- Walking a couple times a week for 20 or so minutes. You're not power walking, but you're able to go longer and probably speedier than last week.

- Changing your child's diaper with only the shadowy light of a nearby bathroom to guide you. (Your diapers have probably downsized to mere over-the-counter maxi pads by now.)

- Fitting into your running hat and shorts. Although the shorts, hugging your thighs and stretched to capacity around your waist, aren't really fit for human consumption. The hat, though, is your new staple accessory: It hides the fact you haven't showered in a week.

What You May Be Concerned About

"My running friend, fresh off a workout, just stopped by to see the baby. I was still in the PJs I've been wearing for 48 hours. Do you think she noticed my stench?"

A maternal odor—a mix of copious sweat, monster breath, sour milk, and foul pads—is nothing to be embarrassed about. It just shows you're concentrating on the task at hand! While she may have felt a jolt from your pits when you gave her a hug, don't worry: The scent she'll recall from the visit is that unmistakable blend of warmth, innocence, and spit-up that can only come from a new baby.

6 TO 9 WEEKS
What You Will Probably Be Doing

- Avoiding telling your husband you got the green light from your doc at your 6-week post-partum checkup to have sex. You're pretty sure you'd rather run a marathon. Barefoot. Over broken glass.

- Laughing when your doc says she wants to talk about birth control. Has she even been listening to your tales of 2-hours-of-sleep nights and an inconsolable baby? That's all the birth control you'll need for now, thanks.

- Suppressing the urge to strangle a woman from church who you, on a rare solo errand, run into at Target and she asks when you're due.

- Making an appointment to get your bird's-nest hair styled. Thanks to plummeting estrogen levels, the Breck-commercial hair you sported during pregnancy is no longer: You're shedding about 100 hairs daily, as your clogged shower drain can attest. And your running hat, you're finally realizing, isn't doing you any favors.

- Loving how forgiving the elastic bands on your running shorts are.

- Jamming to your running mix as you clean the house and fold laundry.

What You Will Possibly Be Doing

- Taking a maiden voyage. Go slowly, go without expectation, walk as often and as long as you need to. After getting home in one piece, reward yourself with a DVD you've been wanting to see, an extra-long shower, or a pedicure.

- Buying an industrial-strength sports bra after your maiden voyage.

- Second-guessing the nurse's skills when you see your weight at the checkup. Turn around on the scale if you think you'd be better off not knowing. (And repeat after me: "9 months on, 9 months off.")

- Remembering to do Kegels when you're standing in a grocery store line or stopped at a light. The leaking, which happens when you sneeze, laugh, cough, run, or otherwise move suddenly, must be stopped.

What You May Be Concerned About

"I used to have everything dialed: up at 6, head out for a run, home, shower, work, home by 6, maybe a yoga class, dinner, bed. Now the only thing I can count on is total disarray. I wasn't expecting a robot, but this baby has no sense of day or night, or how long a proper nap is. I plan to get up to run, and he needs to be fed. I decide not to run, and he sleeps in too. When will he get the memo?"

I remember spending entire days in my running garb, waiting for a chance to pounce. It often didn't come, so I'd recycle the outfit, stained with burp and milk, and try it again the next day. Unable to get my ya-ya's out, I felt resentful toward my baby, who, fortunately, didn't have a clue; my due-at-the-office husband, who did have a clue; and running, with which I had a very dependent relationship. Babies do eventually develop a rhythm, but don't count on it to jibe with the one from your former life.

In the meantime, come up with a list of acceptable Plan Bs for times when you can't hit the road: a yoga video (sun salutations build buff arms for hauling around those 2-ton car seats), a new mom friend to babysit (she brings her infant to your house, you run, then she runs while you watch the two), a home strength routine (see page 110), and an attitude that accepts the quirks and roadbumps of loving a being who knows nothing but to live in the moment—a refreshing and helpful perspective.

3 TO 6 MONTHS
What You Will Probably Be Doing

- Researching jogging strollers. You may be running a couple times a week now, and you want your Plan B to be the same as Plan A: run. Before you go, check with your pediatrician to make sure your kidlet has enough neck strength to withstand your striding; a reclining seat helps soften the blow. As you shop, look for a fixed front wheel and large rear wheels: The bigger the wheels, the smoother the ride will be. Twenty-inch wheels are supreme; 16-inch ones also work well, but 12-inch ones are best left for zoos and malls. Decent protection from the sun, a comfortable handlebar height for you, solid straps and buckles for the baby, and storage for sippy cups for both of you are also must-haves.

- Trying not to twist your ankle when you step off a curb. Relaxin, that helpful hormone that allowed your pelvis to spread so you didn't split in half during birth, is still hanging around in your blood, causing all your joints to continue to do some, um, relaxin'.

- Wondering whether you'll ever get your abs back. Not without work, say the realistic but often cold *What to Expect* experts: "For most women . . . returning the abdomen to prepregnancy tone will require more than waiting for time and nature to take their course. In fact, it will sag for a lifetime unless a concerted effort is made." In other words, when your baby lies on her playmat, get on your back too and crunch away.

What You Will Possibly Be Doing

- Entertaining the idea of doing a 5K fun run with some friends. Emphasize the fun: Run/walk as a group, then head out for brunch or rehydrate with margaritas.

- Shimmying into your pre-preggo jeans. You're likely to have dropped at least 25 pounds by now, and maybe even more if you're running regularly. You may not feel like a rock star when you run, but the word *blimp* doesn't cross your mind anymore when you study yourself post-shower.

- Questioning your commitment to being a runner. After a sleepless night—and there are still plenty of those—running sounds about as appealing as having your in-laws move in with you.

TAKE IT *From* A MOTHER
WHAT WAS THE HARDEST THING ABOUT POST-PREGNANCY RUNNING?

"My gigantic boobs. There isn't a sports bra out there that can accommodate the sheer torque of triple Ds full of liquid."

—KYNDRA (will never run a marathon because "anything that causes your toenails to fall off or your nipples to bleed sounds like a clear message from nature to me.")

"I nursed before I left the house, but then I'd worry about if the baby was crying while I was out running, which, of course, made my milk let down while I was running."

—MOLLY (best part of racing: pushing myself, the swag, the rush from a big event.)

"C-section + no sleep + work = a very grumpy and out-of-shape mom."

—TAMI (longest run in one stint: 30 miles.)

"Getting over the guilt that something or someone—older kids, infant, husband, laundry—should be taking that priority spot."

—KAREN (never warms up or cools down. "I know it will haunt me one day.")

"My stomach would cramp up on me a lot easier than it used to. I think the muscles were still weak; I didn't realize how much you use your abs for posture while running."

—ASHLEY (longest run: 15 miles so far, but training for her first marathon.)

"Getting motivated to run. Most of the time I wanted to use my free time to sleep. Also, my body felt so different, and it was hard to not fit into any of my running clothes."

—CHERYL (favorite cross-training: boot camp.)

"The bouncing. My body was blubber, things that never shook before made me feel like a huge blob."

—MELANIE (running gear peeves: clanking zippers, bouncing hoods, or anything she has to pull up or down.)

> *"I was so out of shape after not having run for about 10 months. But what was hardest were the aches and pains I had 'down there.' I could've sworn my uterus was going to fall out."*
>
> —AMY (ends her Saturday long runs at Dunkin' Donuts. "It's part of the workout.")

What You May Be Concerned About

"I've seen flocks of moms out together, all pushing strollers and gabbing away as they lunge across a park during a Stroller Strides class. I never pictured myself as a mom's group kind of mom, a woman who befriends other women simply because we have kids the same age. But now I want to join them. Is it lame for me to compromise my friendship standards?"

There are the fantasies you create while the kid is still in your belly—a movie-worthy birth, a pacifier-free existence, an undemanding kid—and then there's reality: an emergency C-section delivers a tyke who needs one paci in his mouth and one in each hand to fall asleep. Ditto with friendship expectations. You think you'll keep your circle of friends tight, but after Mr. Plastic-Sucker rears his head, your single friends drift and your mom friends with older kids are too busy to hang.

Time for a reality check: Don't be a friend snob. You can still have your soulmates with whom you do regular drinks–dinner–movie dates, but you can also find the casual pals with whom you laugh, in between curbside calf raises, about the mundane details of your daily life. You don't have to share your life stories, but chances are, you'll at least tell your birth stories—and become close in the process.

6 TO 12 MONTHS
What You Will Probably Be Doing

- Not really noticing, but still appreciating, the rhythm your forever intertwined lives are taking on. You know now that if your kid wakes at 2 A.M., he'll sleep until at least 7:30, so you can run. You know 10 A.M. is the perfect time for you to run for 45 minutes as he snoozes in the baby jogger.

- Not fretting if you miss a scheduled run. You've learned taking time off—whether it's 15 months or one day—just really isn't that big of a deal.

- Trying on your sleekest tank and shorts and checking yourself out in the mirror. *Could I wear these on a run?* Yes.

- Hooking up with your former running group or buddy, if you have one. You now feel confident enough to keep up the pace or go the distance.

What You Will Possibly Be Doing

- Feeling faster than you were pre-babe. Although there's no sound scientific evidence to back it up, reports abound of mothers being swifter than they were when they were child-free. Potential reasons: more oxygen-carrying red blood cells in your body, a higher pain tolerance cultivated through birth, hormonal changes. Honestly, the reason doesn't matter: If it's happening to you, revel in it.

- Contemplating a half-marathon out loud. The whole enchilada sounds like too much to digest, but a couple 12-mile training runs on the weekends feels doable.

- Secretly wondering about a marathon. *If I run a half in 3 months*, you think, *then keep training, could I be ready in 2 more months?*

- Wondering how much you'll be set back when you get pregnant a second time around.

What You May Be Concerned About

"I used to be a really serious runner: I had a periodized, annual schedule, I charted my heart rate and mileage daily, I regularly stood on podiums, there was no such thing as a 'fun' run. Even though I'm still running, I'm not half as interested in it as I used to be. I can't stomach the idea of speedwork, and I haven't signed up for a race because I fear what my finishing time will be. Will I ever get my drive back?"

Maybe, and maybe not. Way back in the day, I heard Oprah, the wise woman and marathon finisher, say you can only do three things really well in your life at one time. Pre-kid, your trio was probably your relationship with your husband, your job, and running. Now, something has to be kicked out to make way for your newest sweetie pie, and it sounds like running is it. When your babe is older, you may be able to sandwich your husband and kid into a "family" package and make room for running. Or you could win the lottery and running can become your job. Until then, do your best to work with your new level of intensity: Trail run, find a group of running moms, steer clear of races. Just as kids go through endless phases, your running has too, and you might enjoy this stage if you give yourself the chance.

.2 IF YOU GIVE A MOM A PAIR OF RUNNING SHOES AND 40 KID-FREE MINUTES*
By Dimity

If you give a mom a pair of running shoes and 40 kid-free minutes, she's going to want to go for a run.

If she wants to go for a run, she'll need to put on a bra—a sports bra, preferably.

When she digs for her bra in a massive pile of dirty laundry, she'll spot her daughter's favorite, must-wear-four-times-a-week starry shirt covered in glitter glue. She'll head to the laundry room to drench the stains in Shout.

As she descends two flights to the basement laundry room, the phone will ring.

When the phone rings, she will check caller ID. She recognizes the number of an annoying mom of a whiny kid who can't seem to grasp the "play" part of "playdate." She lets it go to voicemail.

When she replaces the phone in the jack, she'll remember she didn't charge her iPod. Oh well.

Continuing on to the laundry room, she will decide she should pee before she runs. On the toilet, she will spy another sports bra, hanging on the bathroom doorknob.

When she sees that sports bra, she'll bring it to her nose to see if it's clean or crusty from last week's run. Lucky day: It's clean.

When she heads back up two flights to her room to get dressed, she'll spot a guaranteed no-leak sippy cup, filled with tepid chocolate milk, spouting like a whale on the brand new rug she splurged on at Pottery Barn.

When she sees the brown blob, she'll drop the f-bomb. And then she'll be glad only the dog was around to hear.

After she flies back downstairs to get the carpet equivalent of Shout, she will douse the rug in chemicals not fit for inhalation by dogs or kids. She cracks a window and hopes the stain and smell will be gone by the time she finishes her run.

When she finally gets to her room to get dressed, she'll realize she doesn't remember where she put the bra.

As she runs back down the stairs, her left hamstring will twinge. So she throws her leg up on the kitchen counter and flops toward her toes in a half-hearted attempt at flexibility.

When she stretches her hand around her foot, she will see that her watch reads 2:20, which leaves her exactly 20 minutes for her 40-minute run.

She will swear again, then dart from room to room in search of the bra, get dressed, lace up her shoes, and sprint out the door.

And when she hits the road, she'll wonder why she's out of breath before she even started.

---

*Inspired by the 423 or so times I've read *If You Give a Mouse a Cookie* by Laura Joffe Numeroff.

20

MARRIAGE: **THE SIGNIFICANCE OF THE OTHER**

By Sarah

Husbands fall into two camps: those who run, or do similar sweaty endeavors, and those who don't. How do I know? Because I've had one of each. Yup, that's right, a fact about me even my own kids don't know yet: I had a different husband before I married their dad.

Jack, the cute, quick-witted, warm-hearted man I'm married to now and the father of my three kids, is hubby #2 for me. Hubby #1, charming and sensitive, was named John. To confuse matters, John is also the name of my son, but he's named after Jack, whose real name is John. So, really, I've been married to two Johns and given birth to one. Got it straight?

I don't want to call Jack a couch potato because the term is so hackneyed. Instead, let me tell you that when we first met, Jack's blue-and-green plaid sofa had a deep gully smack dab in front of his TV, which was eternally tuned to ESPN. (Early in our dating life, silly me asked him, "Is *SportsCenter* a channel?" because the show seemed to be on a continuous loop.) John, on the other hand, had been the captain of the men's rowing team in college the same year I was head of the women's crew. We started running together in college, and we kept it up for the rest of our relationship.

With John, because we were kid-free, we always ran together before work. We'd trot about 6 miles through the Presidio when we were in San Francisco or along the Charles River after we moved to Beantown, chitchatting about our lives. Articles I was writing, his clients, a movie we had seen, or what restaurant we'd go to that night. We'd even talk about ridiculous outfits other runners were sporting or women runners in need of more supportive sports bras. (Don't call him a pig: I, not John, always instigated that topic.) Our pace was evenly matched, and John was always agreeable about whatever route I suggested. The miles and the minutes passed quickly, and they are some of my favorite memories of my first marriage.

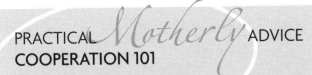

PRACTICAL *Motherly* ADVICE
COOPERATION 101

By Dimity

Although Grant enjoys an hour or three of ESPN as much as Jack does, he also likes to sweat almost as much as I do. Exercise is like a toy both our kids are yanking at; somebody can play with it now, somebody has to wait to play with it later. We don't have a secret formula for working out our athletic schedules. We generally just alternate, both with daily training and bigger goals. These days, for instance, I have mornings on Monday, Wednesday, and Friday to do what I want, and he has Tuesday and Thursday mornings. I get three days because he has the potential for lunchtime workouts during his work week, which I don't. For weekends, we generally talk on Friday about what we want to do, and we either split up the days or make a plan. For example, I run Saturday morning, home by 8:30, he rides at 9, home by 11; switch it up for Sunday.

Same with races: We can't both be training for something epic at the same time. Speaking from experience, two physically fried, mentally tapped parents don't translate to anything close to a healthy home environment. So I take a turn, training for a triathlon while he goes into maintenance mode, then he signs up for a 50-mile mountain bike ride and I dial it back.

Sometimes I feel a little shortchanged, especially when he doesn't heed the (informal, unwritten) rules and starts training for something before I'm officially done. And I'm not afraid to tell him so. "I still get precedence," I remind him as he secretly tries to ramp it up. I take it as a compliment: I'm so excited for my event, he can't wait to pop his cork. More importantly, I miss him. We pretty much fell in love riding our bikes, so when I'm on a solo bike ride, I often wish I were watching his skinny ankles pedal in front of me. Our "date night," when I'm organized enough to put one together, is often on a Saturday morning, traveling over 40 miles of pavement.

This all comes across much smoother on paper than it is in reality. Just because a spouse is physically present and not exhausted doesn't necessarily translate to a parent who is super-attentive to the needs of the house and the family. After a long run, I want more sympathy (read: the floor swept, my back rubbed) during the day, and I imagine he wants the same after an epic ride—or at least an hour to meticulously clean his bike in peace. Instead, my mom-switch gets flipped on as soon as I step back inside the house, and I, forehead still glistening and quads still shaking, am often emptying the dishwasher and coloring pictures of butterflies before I shower or even eat. As imperfect as the system is, I console myself by thinking we're setting a good example for our kids, through both our sweat sessions and playing fair.

TAKE IT *From* A MOTHER
DO YOU RUN WITH YOUR HUSBAND?

"When I started training for my first marathon, my husband, also a non-runner then, and I ran around the same track. We quickly learned this does not work. He's much faster than me. He used to smack my butt with his hand as he lapped me. So, yes, I like to run alone."

—KAMI (a yoga devotee for 20 years. "I love to be flexible; stretching is dessert for me after a difficult workout.")

"If my in-laws are in town or we have somebody to watch the boys, we will sneak away for a quick run. Those times are few and very cherished. My husband is my training partner regardless if he is on a run with me or not. He supports me 110 percent. I couldn't run strong mentally or physically without him."

—MELANIE (first runs: 3-milers in the basketball off-season with Gonzaga teammates.)

"Sometimes. He's 6 foot 5 and I'm 5 foot 3. Those long legs are killer to keep up with."

—KELLY (favorite run: to the top of Mount Tabor in Portland, Oregon.)

"No. He's a builder, so he gets plenty of exercise on the job. He's my biggest supporter, though, and loves to cheer me on at races. He's even volunteered at several of them."

—ANGIE (sign daughter held at a marathon: "Run Like You Stole Something!")

"No, but we go to a park and take turns running while the other plays with the kids."

—CHRISTINE (most memorable race: 2006 Philadelphia Distance Run. "I needed a dose of personal accomplishment at that time, and the race certainly offered it.")

"On occasion. We met at the Hood to Coast, and I thought he had a great interest in running. Turns out, he's just a really talented athlete without much effort. The last time he told me he wanted to get into a running routine with me, I was 12 weeks pregnant. Nice timing."

—MEGAN (best part of running: "It is consistently good, just for me, and never gets old.")

"Occasionally he will go with me part of the way, and I'll push the stroller. But most of the time he doesn't because he can't keep up with me, and I get annoyed if I have to slow down."

—IVANA (p.s.: "When I am in a bad mood, my husband will say, 'Just go for a run. Please.'")

"Yes! He pushes our two kids in the stroller and is very supportive of me. He helped me get a PR in Portland's Race for the Roses and stuck with me during a challenging race at the Seattle Rock 'n' Roll Marathon. I wouldn't have finished at all if he hadn't helped me through the last 8 or so miles."

—MONICA (also loves to run with Kenai, her golden retriever.)

"Sometimes, but he likes to talk and joke around, and I like to zone out. Plus, he usually ends up running ahead of me or pushing the pace, both of which bug the crap out of me."

—TINA (Ironman husband is good for inspiration. "I tell myself, if he can race 120 miles, I can finish a 20-mile training run.")

Most of our individual runs tend to blur together in a happy montage, but to this day when I navigate a city street corner on a run, I often still think of John, who often quoted his high school ice hockey coach during our outings. "Cut corners in practice, you cut corners in a game," he'd remind me. "Cut corners in a game, you cut corners in life." While we were together, John struggled to live up to his potential—the weight of the world often seemed too heavy for him—so this was a bittersweet mantra for him to have. I'll always have a soft spot in my heart for John, and this phrase still speaks volumes to me about him.

When our marriage broke up unexpectedly (to me, anyway), I was bereft of a running partner as well as a life partner. Both were tough losses, so I daydreamed about replacing both of them by meeting a super-sporty guy, someone with even more get-up-and-go than I have. Oh, yeah, and I also wanted him to be a few years younger than I was—maybe 5 or 6 years—so that he wouldn't predecease me. Gotta think long term! An amateur mountain bike racer, for instance, who would rouse me at 7 A.M. on a Sunday to do a 3-hour ride in the Marin Headlands. Or a triathlete who'd suggest run–bike–run "brick" workouts we could do together. I actually went on a few dates with a marathoner, and I started envisioning us running together with our chubby-cheeked firstborn in a jogging stroller.

And then I met Jack. A guy who had last sprinted while trying to catch the El on his way to work in downtown Chicago. A man who actually preferred 20-yard pools to 25-yard ones because it meant he got to rest on the side of the pool more often. A fellow who knew every sports bar in Chicago and which teams' fans frequented them but who had no clue who marathon legends Bill Rodgers or Joan Benoit Samuelson were.

One warm day in April, about 5 months into our courtship, Jack and I decided to go for a run together on the path flanking Lake Michigan. I don't remember which one of us suggested it, but we were both willing participants. Or so I thought. We ran side by side, heading north along the lakefront. I had to slow down to not outpace him, but I didn't mind. It was a blue-sky day, and I was once again running with a man I loved. At least for 20 minutes. Then Jack stopped at a water fountain and said, "You go ahead. I prefer to run alone."

I took his words at face value and chugged ahead. I mean, I appreciate alone time when I run, too. A few weeks later, I told this story to a bunch of work buddies, and this guy Mike blurted out, "Yeah, I use that same excuse when I am being outgunned by a woman." Oh. It had never dawned on me Jack was trying to save face by finishing the run alone.

Needless to say, that was our one and only run together.

Years have passed, and we now have three young children. *SportsCenter* isn't on the endless loop it once was, Jack has gotten moving by shooting hoops with the kids, but I'm running more than ever now. Like so many mommies, I run on weekdays while the rest of the clan is still deep in sleep. But on the weekends, I head out after the sun has risen, and it leads to resentment. Our main sticking point: Mass. Jack goes, I don't. During marathon training, when my runs surpass 2 hours, he goes to church at 7 A.M., then I go running immediately when he gets back. On the days he opts to sleep in—as is his right—then he's stuck either skipping Mass or taking all three kiddos along to 9 A.M. services. He forgoes church about as often as the foursome hits it together. I've never been with them, but I know the ordeal involves sitting in the "cry room" the entire time and trying to keep preschooler Daphne from hitting other kids. Oh, yeah, and bribing them with promises of being able to light a candle afterward—and blowing it out, of course. Something tells me Jack has to squelch the twins' attempts to sing a rousing rendition of "Happy Birthday" in the vestibule.

When I'm not in marathon mode and can scale back my long runs, we settle into a third alternative: I head out at 7 but get back by 8:45, in time for him to dash to 9 A.M. Mass. Jack gets to sleep in *and* visit with his Maker on a weekly basis. This way, I figure I'm getting in his good graces for my next round of marathon training. (For the record, Sundays are my long run day because Saturday morning is when my rowing team practices.)

I realize my Sunday runs are an imposition to Jack, and even though I don't practice anymore, I'm Catholic enough to feel guilty about it. I usually try to circumvent a confrontation about Sunday morning scheduling by discussing it in advance rather than springing it on him at the last minute. Still, every few months, Jack lets me know he doesn't like me eating up a chunk of time on what could otherwise be a lazy family morning. Unlike a lot of moms I've talked to who regularly remind their husbands their sanity is tied to their mileage, I haven't yet vocalized to Jack that no one would be happy in the house if I skipped my run; by midday I'd be blowing my spout more often than Old Faithful. Maybe because I'm not sure he'd grasp the sanity-saving premise.

Instead, I take it upon myself to carry the load for the rest of the weekend. I take the kids to the park or the science museum, leaving Jack with what I consider the ultimate luxury: a quiet, deserted house. I make dinner both nights, then I herd our three cats from PJs to toothbrushing, book reading, and lights out.

Most of the time I don't feel resentful. I actually feel fortunate because other than church, I don't have anything else to conflict with my weekend workouts. Since we're not a two-jock household, Jack and I don't need to juggle my runs with his bike rides or golf games. The only sports Jack cares about are on TV, and the kids can always join him in watching a Kansas City Chiefs game (or they can trash the house while he's intent on touchdowns and turnovers, as usually happens).

But you know what does bug me about this arrangement? Often Jack doesn't seem appreciative enough of having a runner wife and all the benefits that go with it. Having a wife who weighs the same after having three kids as she did when we first started dating. (Actually, come to think of it, a few pounds less.) Or one with slender legs toned by countless miles and hill repeats. And a sparky attitude fired up most days by conquering a run. I know Jack is impressed by my running accomplishments—and the physique and temperament they have produced—but usually he's too blasé to comment on them.

I have discovered one surefire, running-related way to get his attention, though. Jack should say a prayer of thanks at church to the running skirt. Because I want to stay, um, well groomed, I get a bikini wax every so often, especially during skirt season (the skirts I favor have underwear-like "spankies" underneath). When I'm freshly waxed, it just takes mere mention of that fact—let alone a glimpse of the new landing strip—and Jack thinks having a runner for a wife is the greatest thing since, well, *SportsCenter*.

Maybe even better.

.2 HORIZONTAL SWEAT SESSIONS
By Sarah

When I was training for my latest marathon, my coach, Lynn, gave me all sorts of recommendations. Relax my arms. Take an iron supplement. Skip hosting book group if I was stressed. And have sex with Jack.

Yup, unlike collegiate coaches who forbid their wrestlers from getting busy before a big meet, my coach occasionally urged me to hop on Pop. She doesn't believe having intercourse improves running speed or endurance, but she wisely knew attending to my husband's desires on a Friday night would make him all the more agreeable for 3 hours of kid duty on Sunday morning while I trotted 20 miles.

Lynn and I laughed whenever she mentioned it, but I dutifully followed her instructions, even when I was irked at Jack for walking away from dirty dinner dishes or when my whole body cried out for bedtime, not sacktime. Going at it with Jack was always an excellent suggestion. And not just for his sake. Sex is one of those things I often forget how much I like, until I'm in the act. In that respect, it's kind of like running: I can feel drained and disinterested, but once I get going, I'm ohhh-so-glad I took the plunge.

Alas, I won't have Lynn to guide me through my next marathon, but I'll take away this training tip: Always include some intimate cross-training.

21

CHILDREN: MANAGING THE OFFSPRING

By Dimity

There are two ways my kids relate to my running.

Way one: They hate it.

When I change into my running clothes, Ben, who is looking at a machine book on the bed, says, "Mom? Are you going running?" I whisper, "Yes," and he goes back to examining street sweepers. Meanwhile, Amelia, who was happily chatting to her dolls in her room 5 seconds ago, suddenly streaks into the bedroom. "MOM! DON'T GO!" she screams as she leeches onto my quad and forces tears from her ducts. Never mind she might have spent the next 45 minutes—the amount of time I'm planning to run—in her room, oblivious to my absence. Never mind we spent 12 full hours together yesterday, and today, after this quick run, we've got another full day planned. Never mind I've gone for a run at least 1,000 times in her 6 years of life, and every single time, I return.

Doesn't matter. She acts like I'm going on a 6-month trip to Turkmenistan. Her histrionics usually tip Ben over the edge too, and he crawls off the bed and commands the other leg. "Grant, can you help me please?" I yell to my absent husband, unaware that he's parked on the can. His lack of response sets off my impatience, so I take matters into my own hands. I extricate my legs from the octopus arms, cruise down the stairs, and focus my eyes on the prize: the front door. I open it a crack, slip out to the wails of, "Mom! MOM-MA!" and don't look back. I'm surprised my neighbors haven't called Child Protective Services on me yet.

It goes without saying that when I finish, the pair, perched in front of the tube, doesn't even acknowledge my return.

Way two: They want to be like me.

TAKE IT *From* A MOTHER
WHAT'S THE MOST MEMORABLE THING
YOUR KID HAS SAID ABOUT RUNNING?

"When I was 9 months pregnant with my second son, I was sitting on the couch like a beached whale, watching all these svelte, super-fast women running the 5K in the Olympic Trials. My toddler pointed to the TV and said, 'Look, there's Mommy! Go, Mommy, go! Run faster!'"

—CARMEN (follow her at backfrombaby.blogspot.com.)

"We had to take our preschooler to the ER for stitches in her finger. Even weeks after the stitches were removed, she refused to let us cut off her neon green hospital ID bracelet. Why? 'It just makes me run faster,' she said."

—SUSAN (went from being the chubby kid with asthma in eighth grade to finishing a 100-miler at age 42.)

"When I came home from the Boston Marathon, my son asked if I won."

—SHERI (fastest marathon: St. George, which she dedicated to her father, who was dying of cancer.)

"My 5-year-old proclaimed she was going to run a marathon like Mom and Dad. So she's running a mile a day on the treadmill for 26 days. She's already run 10 miles, although she said her seventh day was her 'rest day.' She requires water and 'nutrition' for every run."

—JUNKO (favorite treadmill workout: intervals. "I secretly love running full throttle while the guy next to me is plodding along. Girl power!")

"When my kids were in the stroller, my favorite lines were, 'Faster, Mommy, faster!' and 'More bumps! I like that!'"

—TINA (running helps me focus and process. "Like meditation with a cardio bonus.")

"My 6-year-old is like a little coach. When I was on the bike trainer, doing a Spinervals DVD with hill intervals, he was intently watching the television screen, which had an effort meter. Then he said, 'Are you really working at 100 percent? Because if you're not, you may as well get off the trainer and let Daddy try.'"

—RAQUEL (best part of running: spending time inside my head.)

> *"I was pushing my daughters in a 5K. Right after we took off, several runners passed me immediately and one daughter turned and said, 'Oh, you lost, Mom!' I said, 'Turn around, look at how pretty the course is, and let Mommy run, OK?' What a downer: 20 yards into a 5K!"*
>
> —MARY (note to self: "Do not eat spicy barbecued shrimp the night before a marathon.")

When she was 4 years old, Amelia ran one race, the Scream Scram, around Halloween. Dressed as a butterfly, she ran the 100 meters as fast as she could, her antennae bobbing along. Afterward, she couldn't stop talking about it—and the giftbag. She hung her race number on her door. The following Monday, Ms. Jenny, her preschool teacher, told me she'd never seen Amelia so proud as when she recounted the race for her.

For the past 2 years, I've been meaning to sign her up for another fun run but simply haven't gotten around to it. Still, Amelia orders me regularly to watch how fast she can run or to say, "Ready, set, go!" as she and Ben race across the lawn.

The Jekyll/Hyde scenarios strike signature feelings of parenthood: guilt and pride. The former is easy to summon. Just think of that training adage, "Somewhere out there, somebody is working harder than you are," and you pretty much have parenting in the uber-ambitious twenty-first century in a sentence. Somewhere out there, a mom spends Saturday morning hovering over her first-grader doing addition tables, schlepping her kid to tae kwon do lessons, organizing a neighborhood playdate for five kids at her house, or patiently making blueberry muffins with him and not getting angry when the new bag of flour spills all over the floor.

Somewhere out there, a mom is not running. That mom is not me. I typically don't feel like I should be reading *Frog and Toad All Year* for the fifth time in 2 days instead of doing a tempo run. But I'm not immune to twinges of maternal guilt. As relief fills my body when I run down the block, out of my kids' formidable vocal ranges, I do wonder: Will their early memories of me be dominated by an image of my back, heading out the door, as they scream bloody murder? I doubt it, but it's always a possibility. Memories are so random. I remember things vividly from my childhood—things that have shaped the person I am, I believe—that my two sisters can't even recall, and vice versa. There's no guarantee which of my actions will stick to their souls and which will bounce off.

Then Amelia busts out a race like the Scream Scram, and any guilt I feel is replaced by a ridiculous amount of pride. Rosy cheeked, she held my hand, swinging it back and forth as we walked back to the car. I'd trade mastering reading's silent "e" any day for a moment like that.

Maternal guilt seems to be inversely proportionate to the child's age. The younger the kid is, the guiltier you feel for leaving him. When you walk out the door, unsure if your wailing 2-month-old will take a bottle of freshly pumped milk, your heart weighs heavy. When you walk out the door, certain your 6- and 3-year-olds will stop their dramatics in approximately 15 seconds, your heart kind of laughs. And when you walk out the door, leaving behind a moody, monosyllabic 13-year-old who is driving you crazy, I'm guessing your heart wonders if it's fit enough to run for 3 hours, not 1.

I also think guilt subsides when you accept that the time you spend alone running—time spent strengthening your spirit, confidence, and spunkiness—is far more valuable than simple kid face time. As any cubicle jockey could tell you, the amount of time you're at the job is no indication of the amount of time you're actually working. Plus, running is actually a very practical thing to do for a mother who is interested in keeping an even-keeled house. The miles defuse frustrations, create mental order, instill calmness, and reignite flames barely flickering. Delicious memories of my kids and husband often come to me randomly during a run, and they help me remember why I am where I am in life.

After a run, I'm much more willing to spend time rolling trains around a wooden track for 30 minutes with Ben than I would be if I hadn't run. With no run, I become both antsy and ditzy. I half-empty the dishwasher, then half-read an article in the paper, then half-help Amelia put away her laundry, then play with trains for 3 minutes before I remember I have to go send an e-mail I've half-composed. Then the kids get frustrated because I mutter, "Just a minute," to their countless requests for my time or help, and the house turns into a pressure cooker. Until one of us—usually me, I'm sad to admit—blows.

Though I may be home with the kids, I'm often not present for them.

My mom wasn't a runner. Her preferred sweaty outlet during my childhood was the Jane Fonda Workout. I can picture her now in our basement, wearing a black leotard, black tights, and rainbow leg warmers, doing fire hydrant leg lifts. She did have her own version of running, though: horses. During my childhood, we boarded up to five horses in our battered red barn. She stacked their hay, cleaned their tack, and chopped out their water buckets when the Minnesota winters turned them to ice. (Or, more accurately, sent me to do it, but at least she was on top of the chore.) She guided my older sister's very successful hunter/jumper career, and she let my younger sister trot around on Gayland, a pony, for hours on end. Her professional life was also dominated by horses. At various points in her life, she co-owned The Horse Habit, an equipment store; ran multiday horse shows; and, when my parents divorced, got a full-time office job at the local track.

I hated horses. I don't think I ever screamed, "Don't go!" when she went off to ride, but I never enjoyed throwing my leg over a thousand-pound beast and letting it canter off. I can now appreciate horses, though—and not just because I last chopped an ice bucket over 25 years ago. In an indirect way, they taught me how to be a runner. My mom demonstrated how to be passionate about something, how to delicately weave an activity into your life so that it marks you but doesn't define you. She showed me you can be a mother, have another job, and still carve out time for yourself. Although your kids might resent your absence some days, you taking time to run or ride actually teaches them that the world—news to them?—doesn't revolve around them.

Her most lasting lesson, though, was that some of the deepest, truest friendships form through sport. Debbie, my mom's best friend, whom she met at the local barn, drifted a bit after my parents divorced and we sold our horses. Nearly two decades later, Debbie was losing a long battle with multiple sclerosis and Lou Gehrig's disease, and she and my mom picked up exactly where they left off. In between my mom driving Debbie to the dentist for a mouth guard so she could talk, massaging her clawed fingers, and completing other emotionally daunting tasks, the two laughed as hard as they did when they hung out in a horse trailer at the end of a long day, drinking Diet Cokes and gossiping.

I've done this mothering thing for long enough to know that what I want for my kids has little bearing on what they actually want to do. When I'm intent on us all going to the pool, they want to paint. When I'm ready to set up the easel, they've moved on to setting up the Slip 'n' Slide. As every parent quickly learns, "force" is not a verb that works well with kids. Still, I'm going to, um, strongly encourage them to find their own version of running, something that alternately challenges and calms them, makes them feel alive and proud, and surrounds them with lifelong friends.

When this strategy inevitably fails, I'll turn to the other two signature emotions of parenthood: hope and faith. I'll hope they stumble into their version of running, as I did into mine. In the meantime, I'll have faith in the all-to-accurate message from a magnet my mom surreptitiously stuck on my fridge: "Sooner or later, every daughter becomes her mother."

.2 THINGS I'VE LEARNED FROM . . .
By Dimity

MY KIDS

♀ Go all out or don't go. There is no such thing as long, slow endurance pace.

♀ The best kind of race is the kind with a prize at the end.

♀ Don't fret your shoe choice: You can run in bare feet, Crocs, Mary Janes, flip-flops. But if you're in tie shoes, be obsessive about the bow tie. Make sure the rabbit goes solidly through the hole and you've double knotted.

♀ There is no shame in wetting yourself unexpectedly.

MY DOGS

♀ Keep your nose open to possibilities. If you get an intriguing whiff—or view—stop and take it in, because it may not be there tomorrow.

♀ There is never a bad time to run.

♀ Running is best done in packs, or at least in pairs.

♀ The mere sight of a pair of running shoes should be enough to get your tail wagging.

♀ When you get too hot, let your tongue hang out a bit.

♀ Squatting by the path is acceptable.

♀ A leash—whether it's real or an I-can't-do-this virtual one—will only hold you back.

♀ The best recovery from a run is a nap in the sun.

MY (ANNOYINGLY PATIENT AND SMART) HUSBAND*

♀ If your body is hurting before a run, walk for the first part. If it still hurts, go home.

♀ Be methodical. He's completed marathon training plans, including 22-mile runs, without having entered a race just so he can improve and monitor his improvement. His eventual goal: a 3:20, in order to qualify for Boston, which I'm positive he'll reach in about 3 years.

*These lessons, which he really applies, have been hardest for me to learn.

♀ For the first few weeks back from a longer break, concentrate only on turnover, or how many steps you take in a minute. Aim for 90 to 100 steps on each foot; count the number of times your right foot lands in 20 seconds, multiply by 3, and then double that number. (He filled me in on this after I was told to change my running style to shorter, swifter steps. "I've been doing that for years," he said. "I can't believe you write about running and don't do that.")

♀ Don't fret about not running on vacation, over holiday break, or when you're immersed in building a Lego alligator.

♀ There are things way more important than running. My grandmother's funeral was the same weekend as his entry to the Chicago Marathon, and he immediately canceled his plans without a complaint.

♀ Know there's always Plan B. Ultramarathoner Dean Karnazes's 2006 50 states/50 marathons/50 days tour was passing through Minneapolis exactly the same time we'd be there for the funeral. He joined the pack and ran his 26.2 around the downtown lakes.

22

BREAKS, STRAINS, HURTS, PAINS

By Dimity

For better or worse, I am a crier. Without fail, I tear up at school concerts; somehow seeing Amelia and her friends, all dressed up and looking so earnest and proud, solidifies how quickly the years pass. Show me an abused dog, tell me about your latchkey childhood, mention your sister has breast cancer, and I'm instantly sympathetic and wiping my eyes. And when I'm pregnant or PMSing, I'm guaranteed to gush when I watch the final few minutes of *Grey's Anatomy*, which always features a voiceover about a life lesson.

But what really opens the floodgates, as I've learned too many times, is a running injury. I've had plenty over the past two decades—a bone spur in my big toe, a stress fracture in my heel, four hellishly sprained ankles, IT band syndrome, Morton's neuroma, a bunion bigger than a golf ball, a lower back that goes numb on long runs—and yet despite my numerous opportunities to learn how to cope, the only strategy that works for me is sad, salty tears. Rationally, I know a sprained ankle isn't so bad: It puffs up to a cankle, stays ugly and bloated for a few days, then returns to normal. Not really something to cry over. The world can be a horrible place, with wars, disease, and hatred, and uncooperative ligaments do not register on the universal Richter scale of disaster.

But on my navel-gazing scale, an injury rocks me to my core. First off, it pisses me off that the injury is caused by running, an activity we all agree is good for you. It's not like I chain-smoked my way to an angry iliotibial band or never ate any green veggies and, as a result, got nailed with a stress fracture. I was doing my body and spirit a favor, and like a tantrumming toddler who doesn't have the words, it attacked me. Then there's the actual physical pain, which can sting initially but then settles into a gnat-like level: It's just noticeable enough to be annoying, swarms around endlessly, and is almost impossible to kill.

That niggly feeling promotes a self-fulfilling circle of pity: It reminds me I can't run. Void of endorphins, I crave sugar, so I convince myself that handfuls of peanut M&M's are a perfectly acceptable meal because my non-running self is going to gain 20 pounds anyway. Crashing from the sugar high puts me in a foul mood, made even worse by the constant, achy reminder that I won't be running today or tomorrow or anytime soon, and my hand is back in the yellow 1-pound bag of happiness. The intensity of the cycle increases as the injury fails to heal or as the race for which I was training looms.

And so: tears.

In order to defuse this loaded topic and keep my keyboard dry, I've decided to write this chapter as a (mostly) objective Q&A. Please note: I am as far from a doctor as it gets, so please don't mistake any of this for medical advice.

Q: What causes running injuries?

A: There are two aspects to any run: speed and distance. Jam on either of them like a bongo drum, and you'll pay. Both should be conservatively increased over time. The oft-repeated 10 percent rule—increase your weekly distance no more than 10 percent from one week to the next—is the first injury prevention commandment. The second: For most people, speedwork should be no more than 10 percent of your weekly mileage. If the only math you do these days involves figuring out how much to pay the babysitter, here's an example: You're at 20 miles a week. Two of those should be really fast. Next week, you can go about 23 total, and a little over 2 can be speedy. Don't fret the numbers too much: Most beginner and intermediate training plans, found in books, magazines, or online, follow a safe progression.

Then there are myriad other things that can cause injury, everything from the obvious (a root on a trail run that twists your ankle) to the almost invisible (a 2-millimeter difference in your leg length). The slant of the road's shoulder can screw you up, as can the wrong pair of shoes. A too-long stride can take you down, as can quads that overpower your hamstrings. In other words, like anything that involves moving through the world, getting hurt is always a concern.

What I really mean: You know that spring day, when it's a perfect 60 degrees, the sky is bluebird, the husband has the kids at the zoo, and you're finally coming out of hibernation? Take it easy on that run, and the run after that, and after that. Also, wear out your welcome at a running-specific store. Try on at least five brands of shoes, ask "Why" more times than a 3-year-old does, and run, wearing them, on a treadmill before you buy. Once in your perfect-for-you kicks, change things up as much as possible: Run on both sides of the street, hit the trails, lap the track. And always watch out for rocks, curbs, roots, and anything else that can trip you up.

TAKE IT *From* A MOTHER
HOW DID YOU COPE WITH TIME AWAY FROM RUNNING?

"I drove everyone around me crazy. Fortunately, I was able to cross-train on the Concept II rowing machine and bicycle."

—RUTH ANNE (started running because her husband said, "As fast as you walk, you should start running.")

"Not very well. With young kids, I find it very difficult to cross-train during an injury. I can't just come and go as I please to the gym or pool. It's pretty much running or nothing for me. Ugh."

—JILL (elaboration: "If I'm running, I'm happy. If I'm not, then I'm usually not.")

"I ate a lot and got semi-depressed, but got on the bike and elliptical."

—IVANA (trick to strength training: "Just do it. There's no perfect time to start.")

"I strategize for my comeback. I look at it as time for my body to rest and refuel so I can come back stronger."

—JILL (unwelcome audience: three coyotes as she was squatting in the woods. "I ran as fast as I could after they left!")

"I pouted and cried. My husband rolled his eyes."

—KAT (worst part of running: "When I have to go solo.")

"A stress fracture in my talus bone knocked me out of being able to run the first race I had ever signed up for. I was crazy for a while. I wasn't as nice of a mom."

—JEN (songs that settle her into a steady pace: "Bittersweet Symphony" by the Verve and "Solsbury Hill" by Peter Gabriel.)

"I worried about how I would perform when I jumped into training, but I knew that I needed to give my body time to heal. It all worked out."

—KRISTYN (first race: a local 5K. "I proved to myself that I could do it, and I can do more.")

Even then, the pounding nature of running makes you susceptible to injury. In fact, none of those tips have worked for me. My best guess is that my not-so-runnery physique, coupled with my lackadaisical form and genetically problematic feet, are trying to win a contest for creating the most injuries. They know it's the only kind of running-centric event I could ever win.

Q: What can I do to prevent injuries?

A: As tempting as it is, don't totally tune out during a run. Most running injuries are appropriately called overuse injuries: They materialize through using the exact same muscles in the exact same motion over and over again. One day, on your 4,000th or 54,000th step, you'll feel a serious pain on the bottom of your foot, on the side of your knee, the back of your leg, or anywhere other than your head, really. This pain feels distinctly different than the ugh-don't-make-me-go whine your muscles usually produce at the beginning of a run. It means business. It compromises your rhythm or stride. Do not ignore this pain. Do not think it'll go away in 10 minutes. Do not think, "Today, I'll just finish and then I won't run tomorrow."

The responsible thing to do is stop, get home, RICE (rest, ice, compress, elevate), poke around on the Internet to self-diagnose, and call a few running friends for advice. Then see a doctor if necessary, dutifully comply with the regimen of physical therapy or stretches she prescribes, and completely recover before you start to run, at a conservative pace and mileage, again.

What I really mean: Running has an insidious way of finding any muscular imbalance, tightness, or irregularity and heading right for it, kind of like how a hungry newborn roots around for a nipple. Your left calf is tighter than your right? Lucky day: You get plantar fasciitis, a condition on the bottom of your foot that makes getting up in the middle of the night to pee so painful, you contemplate wearing Depends. You overpronate and have weak abductors? Meet your new friend, piriformis syndrome, which will make your butt writhe in pain when you sit, stand, climb stairs, or pretty much just breathe. Lovely.

If you had all the time in the world—or were on the clock only 40 hours a week—you would take the aforementioned responsible steps when you feel an injury creeping in. If you're a smart mother, you'll at least stop for a few days, ice while you wait for the water to boil for spaghetti, and limit the games of tag. If you're a mother too driven to stop—ahem, not naming names here—you'll be stubborn and pay for it for months and maybe even years.

On the heel of a summer of four triathlons and three running races, I wanted to test my fitness at the Denver half-marathon in October 2008; I'd worked so hard for months, racing 13.1 miles wasn't that big of a deal, I thought, selectively forgetting that I was in pain for most of the summer. Most mornings, I'd get up, I'd start my workout, and my left glute and hip would protest. I willfully ignored them for the first few minutes, and then they warmed up enough to just whimper, not scream. Until the workout was over. Then they roared, and I went through most days feeling like a railroad tie was being driven through my knee. I did run the race, but I had to stop running totally for months after the race. And 8 months later, the injury was still going strong.

At least one of us was.

Q: Should I run in pain?
A: No.

What I really mean: Maybe. One of the most helpful interviews I've ever done in regard to injury prevention was with Bob Wilder, M.D., at University of Virginia's Center for Endurance Sport. His rule: Rate your pain from 1 to 10. If it's a 3 or below, you can keep going. If it ranks above 3, cut it short or dial the intensity back. I sometimes idiotically round the 3 up to a 5 and keep going, but I'm trying to be much more diligent about paying attention to my aches and pains.

Q: Am I alone?
A: No. You're actually in good company. According to Dr. Wilder, 70 percent of runners will experience an injury that requires them to take at least a week off of running.

What I really mean: Yes. Kind of how some women act as if they're the first ones who ever popped out a kid, you'll instantly feel like you're the only person who has ever suffered your particular injury. What's more, in your injured state, you'll see runners everywhere, on routes and in places you've never noticed them before. You'll suddenly notice red-cheeked women in running garb in the grocery store and wonder jealously how far they just ran. You'll study race posters intently, races in which you'd otherwise have no interest, and mentally tally the number of weeks away the race is, and calculate whether you could run it. If you have a regular training group, you'll picture them laughing and trotting along—and not missing you.

Q: What kind of injury is the worst?
A: The kind you're suffering from right now.

What I really mean: I'll take a broken bone over a muscular injury any day. Fractured bones, whose progress can usually be monitored via X-ray, eventually fuse back together and you're basically as good as new. Muscles, on the other hand, and their more wicked cousins, tendons and ligaments, can overstretch, snap, or freeze up, depending on their mood. They seize up when you least expect it. They need to be coddled and soothed by a massage and diagnosed, if possible, through expensive CAT scans. They're tangled up in indecipherable ways: If your calf hurts, it may be linked to fascia in your feet or the tendons in your lower back. And, at least in my experience, they never fully heal. (Sorry to be a total downer; just trying to level with you.)

PRACTICAL *Motherly* ADVICE
HOW TO STAY OFF THE INJURED LIST

The ramifications of being a mother can also translate to injuries. (The benefits just never end, do they?) A few points to keep in mind:

- As you may have guessed, looking at those wretched, pale rivers that traverse your belly and thighs, you stretch during pregnancy. And your ligaments don't just snap back after birth; it takes around 9 months for them to return to their pre-pregnancy state. You're especially susceptible to injury during this time, so take it slow and easy.

- Beware of the consequences of toting around an infant predominantly on one hip. I always used my left hip as my kid-ledge, as I'm right-handed and needed that hand free. My biggest running problems after pregnancy? On my left side, including some issues with my hips being way out of alignment. I have no scientific proof the two are related, but it seems awfully coincidental. And I've heard of other mothers having similar stories: injured seemingly out of nowhere but then, after consideration, linking it back to how they carry their child. As awkward as it may feel, try to rotate hips or hook up the center-lying Baby Bjorn as often as possible.

- Your posture has also probably taken a hit during pregnancy; with a 20-ish-pound beach ball cemented on your belly and throwing off your balance, how could it not? Add in breastfeeding or looking down to coo as you bottle feed, boobs larger than cantaloupes, bending to change the babe and pick her up, and your lower back is probably achy and mad. Concentrate on standing tall when you run, and to build supporting abs strength, crunch like you're crunching for your life.

- Watch out for toys underfoot, especially ones with wheels. Sounds obvious, but I've sprained an ankle twice as a result of stepping on a toy the wrong way—not that there's a right way to step on one.

- It's OK to occasionally put a moratorium on carrying your preschoolers. Sure, your momma's boy wants to be carried everywhere like Sarah's John does, but sometimes her body just needs a break. Yours does, too.

Q: Does my spouse, best friend, co-worker care as much about my injury as I do?

A: No. Sympathy—and some very decent advice—is best found on the Internet. Google your injury and you'll stumble into way too much information, including bits about how exactly the injury is caused, how long you're going to be out, and the best way to heal.

What I really mean: Yes, they obviously care about your well-being, but rambling on about it, especially to a non-runner, is likely to elicit boredom, not empathy. A running injury isn't life threatening; you're probably still walking, emptying the dishwasher, putting together Excel spreadsheets, sneaking pureed veggies into pasta sauce, and otherwise carrying on, albeit probably in a more depressed state than normal. That said, the bigger the evidence of the injury, the more sympathy you'll garner: a big black boot cushioning your stress fracture makes you seem way more injured than a minor limp caused by shin splints.

Q: Why is it so hard to get myself to do the exercises my physical therapist prescribed?

A: It is difficult to find the time to get on the floor and contort yourself in random ways while your kids climb all over you. But find the time: Like most medicines, physical therapy makes you better.

What I really mean: I hate how belittling they can feel. After the Denver half-marathon, I finally made it to a very qualified physical therapist, who dissected my movement patterns and found some massive problems with my hips and pelvis. My first assignment, which was all I was supposed to do for a whole week, was to lie on the floor, keep my bottom half still, and pretend, with my upper half, like I was rolling. Ten to the right, ten to the left. Vary my position and repeat. I just grunted through 13.1 miles less than a week ago, and now my whole workout is forty rolls? Not exactly the adrenaline rush I was looking for.

Their simplicity also belies the amount of time they take. I think, "OK, I'll do my rolls while the kids are in the bath." But then laundry needs to be folded, a fight erupts in the tub, or I just want to call my mom, and another day goes by without the exercises. The only way I can make it a priority—and I do need to put them on the front burner if I want to still be running a decade from now—is to give them the same treatment as I give a run. I set my alarm to get out of the house early. Instead of taking off down the bike path on foot, I go to the Y, where my "exercises" fit in well with the arm circles and toe taps the silver striders are doing.

Q: How do I not lose all my fitness gains while injured?

A: Cross-train. Any activity that doesn't aggravate your injury works: You can ride a bike, swim, do yoga, lift weights, ellipticize, hike, or even run in the pool. Spinning and the StepMill (the stair machine that has actual stairs, not pedals like the StairMaster) seem to give the best bang for the cardiovascular buck, but you can challenge yourself on any piece of equipment if you set your mind to it.

What I really mean: As long as you work hard, you'll barely lose any cardiovascular fitness, although you will lose running-specific strength. After I got a stress fracture in my heel while training for the Nike Marathon, I rode my road bike, in my basement on an indoor trainer, for about 8 weeks. The workouts were tough: Most were at least 75 minutes, and some lasted 2 hours, and all involved some changing of the pace, so I was stressing my heart appropriately. (I was fortunate enough to have a coach who gave me daily workouts and pep talks when I didn't think I could pedal nowhere for another minute.) I definitely didn't love it. But I appreciated the results: Not only did my legs come out from the bike sessions surprisingly strong and fresh, but my mind has never been so psyched to run.

Q: Pool running: really?

A: Yes, really. It's as effective as road running; I've interviewed a number of elite athletes who take a weekly day in the pool to give their joints a break but still work their hearts and lungs. Wearing a flotation belt around your waist or supporting your own body weight, you can do intervals or a tempo run and have the same result as you would if you did it on the road.

What I really mean: No freakin' way. Running nowhere in the pool, with nothing to listen to and nothing, save the pimply teenage lifeguard, to stare at is my version of hell. It's even worse than taking care of a house full of strep throat patients, when your individual case is the worst.

Q: What should I do with myself when I'm injured?

A: Indulge in activities you don't have the energy or time to do when you're running regularly. Sleep late (read: until 7 A.M.), learn how to make popovers, finally put together a baby book for your now 7-year-old, and go on a date with your husband.

What I really mean: Do anything you want, but steer clear of the candy aisle at the store.

Q: How do I deal with the friends in my running group?

A: The biggest appeal of running for many women is the friendships formed through it. When an injury sidelines you, it doesn't hurt only your body. It also compromises your feelings of connectedness and belonging. Don't shut them out of your life. Meet them at your regular post-run coffee stop, invite them over for lunch, or go see a movie with a few of them.

What I really mean: If you can see them without feeling lonely and sad, go for it. My friendships built through running tend to be the most robust, supportive ones I have, and that contact helps at least my soul heal. But be aware you're the elephant in the room—hopefully figuratively, not literally—so open up the topic by inquiring how their running is going. If the conversation drags on to mile-by-mile race recaps or other unnecessary minutiae, ask them to put the brakes on the conversation. They should understand.

If it's (understandably) too hard for you to break up the association between friendship and running, drop your group an e-mail telling them you're on the injured list and you'll be back in touch when you're healthy again.

Q: Is it OK to be annoyed by runners who proudly proclaim they've never been injured?

A: Yes.

What I really mean: Yes. Limp away from them as fast as you can.

.2 THE ROAD I TRAVEL (WHEN I'M NOT INJURED)*
By Dimity

I head out and the warmup begins. I'm going to walk

Just to the end of this street, no—check that—the next block.

I yawn and I stretch, and plod to the spot. Legs: It's time to go.

I'm not kidding. So get moving. I fire up the Nano.

Mile 1 is the worst: a concrete path with a slight uphill.

I pray for a car or red light—any reason to stop—as I will

My creaky bones up the sidewalk and across three roads.

Finally, a highlight: the smell of freshly baked dough.

I'm tasting croissants, doughnuts, and other trans fats. Soon enough, the gravel path hits.

With it, a minor downhill and relief for the hammies, no longer wanting to quit.

Slide under two bridges, where the homeless guys pass the night.

They're still asleep under piles of blankets, so I (try to) keep my feet light.

Pike's Peak, the purple mountain majesty, fills the frame as the blue

Of the sky starts to lighten. Morning is here, and I'm done with mile 2.

The next mile also slants down, paralleling a stream. I imagine its swift

Current is carrying my legs, and they're digging the virtual gift.

Mile 4 hits, and I'm truly floating. I ask myself: Go longer?

I can easily add on a mile or two, and, you know, get stronger.

But no, for today, this is exactly how long I should run.

And plus, what's that line about leaving while the party is still fun?

Pass the skeevy apartments, the firehouse, the dog that never shuts up.

And a new woman returns home, to the kids, the shower, the coffee cup.

It's an ordinary, easy route, but it soothes me so well.

It's the path my spirit needs to trace when everything feels like hell.

Four miles of peace, four miles of solitude, four miles of sweat.

Four miles I will never, ever regret.

*With apologies to Maya Angelou and every other poet with any talent.

23

BODY IMAGE: **THE WEIGHTING GAME**

By Dimity

I hate that, as a 37-year-old, college-educated woman, I can be more concerned about the size of my size 12/14 ass than I am about the guy holding a "Homeless vet with family of four" cardboard sign beside an exit ramp. But I come by it naturally. I'm an American woman who has been brought up in a culture where Hillary Clinton, currently the secretary of state, has been maligned for her fat ankles. In a culture where overweight, balding men rule the big screen but any woman bigger than a size 4 has a hard time getting anything besides a bit part. In a culture where putting a real-life woman—somebody with turkey-gobble triceps or a waist that doesn't hourglass—in a magazine doesn't fly, unless, of course, the story is about how she lost 100 pounds and is now a size 4.

I'll now step off my soapbox. Let me add, though, that I really, truly hate that I have a daughter who, despite my best intentions, will probably examine herself in the mirror for flaws, think her body mass index and IQ are equally significant numbers, and be sure her life would improve if she were only 10 pounds lighter.

Which is why I'm going to force—OK, really strongly encourage—her to play sports. Because the only antidote I know that tempers body obsession is bodies in action. I was in motion through most of my childhood, participating in swimming, softball, tennis, skiing, and, way back in the day, even ballet and gymnastics. I sucked on the balance beam and flew when I swam butterfly, but overall, I was an average athlete. And, actually, I didn't even think of myself as an athlete then. Swatting forehands and trying, in vain, to catch flyballs sent a subconscious signal to my brain, still under construction, that my body was more than an object. My limbs were meant to move, to run, to throw, to swim, to be strong.

In other words, I developed a respect for my body without even knowing I was doing it.

Sports gave me a head start in the often brutal war of self versus body, but I still waged battles daily, spurred by the disparity between how my body looked and how I thought it should look. In middle school, the fact that my trendy Guess jeans were size 32, the biggest ones available, bothered me so much, I cut out the tag. I scrutinized the prom models in *Seventeen* for hours, sure their lives were so much better than mine because they had boobs, skinny legs, and fingernails that weren't gnawed raw. I went on a diet—the only one of my life—composed solely of dry Cheerios. Fortunately, it lasted precisely one day.

Age has brought me some peace with my size, but still I stand on the scale these days far too often. I don't check in with my poundage daily, but I'm on it at least twice a week. Ideally in the morning, when I know my weight will be at its lowest, and ideally, after an early run, when I'm slightly dehydrated.

I didn't use a scale for most of the first 25 years of my life. But Grant owned one, and I stood on it not long after he moved in with me. Because I wanted a reference for that number, I stood on it the next day. And the next and next. And an unhealthy habit formed. I can't remember what my weight was in my late 20s; all I wanted to know is whether the number stayed constant, within 3 or so pounds, from day to day. When it tipped over by, say, 5 pounds, I wasn't sent into an exercise frenzy or a grapefruit diet, but I did ratchet up the self-criticism and mileage and limit my wardrobe to blacks and grays. No way I wanted my unworthy body to stand out.

Even though I'm far from being anorexic, fixating on my weight, as any eating disorder counselor could tell you, is all about control. About being disciplined enough to put the right foods in my mouth, and when I don't, exercising the wrong foods away. When I lose the ability to do the latter, I get caught up in the weight game. Being pregnant—something I had looked forward to since my teenage babysitting days—was much harder than I ever imagined it. Seeing that needle zing way up past 200 pounds, even though 220 pounds was a reasonable weight for a 6-foot 4-inch frame, was devastating. My insensitive, male OB/GYN didn't help matters when he commented on how much weight I'd gained in the eighth month of my pregnancy with Amelia. I replied, doing my best to sound unfazed, "Well, it was my birthday and I ate the whole cake." I cried on the drive home.

Injuries also set me off. I remember reading an interview with a celebrity who was going to have bunion surgery and needed to be off her feet for 6 weeks. She was working out like a madwoman in the weeks before in order to mitigate the upcoming weeks of sloth. Even though I know rationally that's not a sound strategy—running for 30 miles one day and then taking the week off is hardly the same as running 6 miles for 5 days—I thought, *I can totally relate*. When I broke my right wrist, snowboarding for the first time, I was on the exercise bike the next morning at the hotel. I needed to know I could still take charge. And when I shattered my left one, which required surgery, I wish I had known I was going to be out for months. I would've banked some calorie-busting exercise. Instead, I became a bit obsessed, checking my weight almost daily during my months of recovery.

I can live day to day without the scale, though. Trying to sell our house, we put all extraneous stuff in storage in order to make it look like the house was much sleeker than it actually was. The scale, which didn't fit nicely into a bathroom corner, was thrown in a box and stayed there for 4 months or so.

When I saw it sitting in the bottom of the "Bathroom" box at our new house, I immediately took off my shoes and stepped on it. When it settled on 174, an acceptable number for me these days, I was relieved. Months of packing, moving, and all the trillions of details those entail—and not running much—hadn't set me back. I'm ashamed to admit this, but *phew*.

The counterbalance to my weigh-ins, running gives me a similar feeling of control. I pick the route. I determine how hard I'm going to work—and, consequently, about how many calories I'll burn. I decide when to go and when I'm done.

Unlike obsessing about weight, which feels superficial and passive, athletic discipline has an admirable, authoritative presence. I can spot a female athlete from across a room. I'm not talking about her muscular quads, cut biceps, or bike glove tan lines. An athlete—and all dedicated runners, regardless of speed, are athletes in my mind—simply moves through the world in a way non-athletes don't. Some swagger, and some are more quietly secure. Either way, they talk with authority and walk with purpose, suggesting a self-confidence that comes only from hours of sweating and striving. A female athlete sends out a message that she knows exactly what she's capable of—quite a lot, thank you—and that she is, more often than not, comfortable in her own skin.

Although running isn't a sport where your every curve is on stage, like figure skating or gymnastics, it's not exactly curling or archery either. At a race, bodies are on display. Sculpted calves testify to hill repeats, knees in braces tell stories of frustrating injuries. You can tell which runners will lead the pack simply because they have the ideal runner's body: lean, compact, graceful, vibrant. (Or, if you want another clue, just look for who is confidently traipsing around in her bunhuggers.) Contrast that with the women who have decided they'll somehow squeeze the ideal from their non-runner frame. Fly-away hair and raisin-like cheeks, they look so frail, you could snap them. They may be fast today, but next year, they'll probably be a tangle of stress fractures.

Then there's the rest of the field, whose bodies give almost no clue about how they'll run. Quads can be birdlike or bricklike; bellies can be concave or convex. Until the gun goes off, you have no idea

TAKE IT *From* A MOTHER
HOW MUCH OF YOUR RUNNING IS FOR WEIGHT CONTROL?

"A fair percentage. There's always a part of me that believes I can make improvements to my physique one way or another. After a particularly heavy meal, I can't wait to go run it off."

—ANGIE (ultimate benefit of running: coming to a better understanding about the world and people around her.)

"About 50 percent. My family history of heart disease runs deep, so running is my preventive way of staying away from the pharmaceuticals. I come from good Iowa stock, so being lean is not the norm!"

—JESSICA (favorite treadmill workout: 10-minute warmup, bump up the speed every minute until she can't hold the pace, 10-minute cooldown. "Short and sweet!")

"The shorter runs are for weight control. I eat so much before, during, and after a long run that I think it all evens out."

—KAT (most effective strength move: one-legged squats.)

"It's a factor, but it's not about a number on the scale. It's more about keeping my metabolism fired up in my late 30s so that I can continue to eat what I want."

—MAGGIE (hates running shorts with a passion. "I also have a million ideas for the redesign of sports bras.")

"It's not. I love to eat, I like to drink, I love to run. If any one of these three things starts to impact the others, I know I need to readjust."

—JEN (best part of racing: adrenaline, accomplishment, great legs everywhere.)

"It definitely started out as that, but I have grown to love running for running's sake. I do also like the side effect that I can eat most things."

—KIRSTEN (favorite race: Boston Marathon. "It's worth the hype.")

how fast 95 percent of runners are. Case in point: my triathlon coach, Abby, whose lower half looks capable and dense but not particularly fast. Don't be fooled, as Katherine, my running partner, was. "She qualified for Boston?" she asked me on a run. "How?"

In fact, Abby, a six-time Ironman finisher, has qualified for Boston three times and is currently training for the Leadville 100 race, a mere 100 miles at 10,100 feet elevation or above. She is a perfect example of taking what you genetically got and running with it. If you imagine your body as a lump of clay, running is the pottery wheel on which you toss it. The miles caress and squeeze it, but fundamentally, the clay is still the same mass. It's just molded into kick-ass shape.

Just as I forgot those taffeta-clad *Seventeen* models when I was trying to master moguls as a teenager, I'm least concerned with my body when I'm running. Instead of scrutinizing the aesthetics of my muscles, I become intimate with their substance. In motion, I realize my quads, able to split a designer jeans' seam with a single squat, are engineered perfectly; my calves, which look so big poking out from under an eyelet-trimmed skirt, are strong for a reason; my glutes, rounder than a honeydew melon, are the V-8 motor I need for the hills. On a good run, when I'm pretty sure my strides are helping the earth rotate, I don't care whether I'm 200 pounds or 80 pounds. In motion, my body is doing what it was designed to do. My mind is content, thinking about everything except the number on the scale.

On bad runs, when I'm dwelling on the fact I had six chocolate chip cookies for dessert last night, I'm at least grateful my muscles are strong enough to carry me through every 100-calorie burning mile. Afterward, I try my best to not step on the scale to verify the work they did.

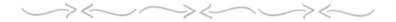

.2 RUT BUSTERS
By Dimity

My freshman year of college, I was rejected by my sorority of choice. I was so mortified, I was ready to catch the next plane home and never return. Instead, the morning after the ax fell, I went to the local elementary school, where I volunteered in the first-grade class. Sitting among low-income kids who were struggling to sound out the word *table,* sucked out of my self-centered pity, I realized being branded by Greek letters wasn't that big of a deal.

You can hit a similar woe-is-me rut in running: You plateau at a certain speed; motivation is harder to find than matching socks in a laundry-folding session; you're just over it. Here are a few of my favorite ways to get over myself.

RELAY

Oregon's Hood to Coast, New Hampshire's Reach the Beach, and Colorado's Get Your Ass over the Pass are runners' versions of raves. Teams are usually made up of twelve runners, with each athlete running three legs of 3 to 8 miles each. Between segments, you'll laugh harder than you have in years, eat Cool Ranch Doritos, blast rowdy music, and get roughly 45 minutes of sleep in 24 hours. If that sounds like your version of hell, consider this: One of my most memorable runs ever was during the Hood to Coast, at 2 A.M., with nothing but the sounds of the night and a full moon to guide my way. (hoodtocoast.com, rtbrelay.com, or wildwestrelay.com; form your own team or join a list of singletons looking for teams on the various sites)

MENTOR

Rediscover the sport through the spindly legs of a 10-year-old. Girls on the Run, a program in more than 150 cities nationwide, is a 12-week, twenty-four-run commitment to share the love with an 8- to 12-year-old girl as you help her train for and run a 5K. You never know: You may be going stride-for-stride with the next Deena Kastor. (girlsontherun.org)

SLICE ORANGES

Or pass out finishers' medals, direct traffic, or refill water cups at a local race. Stale while training for a half-marathon, I signed up to help with the food distribution at the Discover Trail Marathon in Colorado Springs. As I sliced oranges and bananas, I asked every runner who wasn't frowning how his or her race was. The answers I got—"I PR'ed!" to "I made it, but it was hard" to "Never again!"—reminded me you have to embrace the valleys to appreciate the peaks.

SHINE YOUR LIGHT

On the sidelines of a marathon, I'm always in awe of visually impaired athletes who rise to the challenge. Not exactly a graceful athlete who can multitask, I haven't yet been brave enough to volunteer as a guide, but it's on my running bucket list. If you're up for the task, my hunch is your involvement would be more meaningful than any PR ever could be. (achillestrackclub.org)

24

EXERCISE OBSESSION: **ADDICTED TO SWEAT**

By Sarah

Exercise addiction: It's when a good thing goes bad. When your workouts take on a life of their own, crowding out the rest of your life. When running becomes paramount to eating family dinners, going to book club, helping with homework, watching *American Idol,* and even sleeping.

But for many of us, there's a fine line between being committed to exercise and needing to *be* committed. Like me: I didn't think I was addicted to working up a sweat when I exercised every single day for the second half of the 1990s. Yes, every single day for 6 years. But despite how it may sound from the outside and despite many people telling me otherwise, I still don't think I was certifiable.

The Streak, as I affectionately refer to it now, started out innocently enough, as I kept a tally of my workouts on sheets of yellow, lined legal paper. I chicken scratched the date, the workout—"Ran Glen Road loop" or "Exercycle plus Body Pump"—and the length of time it took. I kept the folded sheets stashed in the back pocket of my Franklin planner. One day, killing time at work (who, me?), I perused a year's worth of sheets and tallied how many days I'd missed each month. I realized it was usually only 3 or 4 days each month, so I decided to see whether I could go 1 month straight without missing a workout.

Thus February 14, 1995, became a red-letter date on my workout calendar. That Tuesday stood out not because it was Valentine's Day but because it was the last day on which I didn't exercise for more than 2,000 consecutive days. Which, I now realize, is enough time to have a child progress from being a flailing newborn in a onesie to a first-grader able to write her name and color within the lines.

What qualified as a legitimate workout? Any activity that lasted at least 30 minutes, got my heart rate elevated, and made me sweat somewhat. (And, no, going at it hot and heavy didn't count. So perhaps I should add to the checklist: Wearing workout wear.) I had other rules as well. A walk—

PRACTICAL *Motherly* ADVICE
EXERCISE ADDICTION CHECKLIST

If you have three or more of these symptoms, which are listed in order of severity from fairly harmless to big red flag, you might have crossed the line from devoted to diseased. As with any illness, talk to your physician if you think you have a problem, and she can recommend a therapist.

- You wish Costco sold bigger bottles of ibuprofen.

- You know the number of miles you ran last week, last month, and the last 4 years—and you're happy to tell anyone who will listen about any and all of those runs.

- You dropped out of your synagogue's social committee and stopped coaching your daughter's lacrosse team because both activities cut into your workout time.

- You can't remember the last time you watched TV without simultaneously running on a treadmill, pedaling on a stationary bike, or doing lunges and crunches.

- You haven't had your period in several months, and not because it's time to invest in a double jogging stroller or you're going through perimenopause.

- When you finish a workout, you never feel a sense of accomplishment. Instead, you instantly think about what and when the next one will be.

- You think of running through injuries as another tool by which to increase your mental toughness.

- Your alarm clock is permanently set for 4:30 A.M. because you need to get in a solid 2-hour run before work. You also aim for an hour-long workout after the dinner dishes are done.

- You've left your sleeping, preschool-age kids home alone to sneak out for a run when your husband was away on a business trip because you couldn't bear to miss your daily 8-miler.

gasp—counted as a workout, as long as it was done at a brisk pace and lasted at least 45 minutes. Yet I didn't allow myself to power walk 2 days in a row, just as I couldn't do back-to-back days of strengthening exercises (a half-hour or more of lunges, step-ups, tricep dips, planks, crunches, and

TAKE IT *From* A MOTHER
ARE YOU ADDICTED TO EXERCISE?

"I'm the first to admit I'm addicted to exercise. I place too much emphasis on getting a workout done when other priorities—including those in my best interest—should take precedence. However, I'm a firm believer my running makes me a better mother, wife, employee, friend, human being. I just have to always be sure I keep things balanced."

—ANGIE (follow her at tallgirlrunning.blogspot.com.)

"Oh, totally! If I don't run or work out for a day or two, I'm obsessed with when I can get a workout in. I tend to be a little obsessive overall, and running probably fits into that tendency."

—ALEXA (asked her dad on first run together, "Why does it hurt so badly?" His response: "You're out of shape, kid.")

"No. I love running and start to miss it if I don't run for a few days, but nothing obsessive."

—BRANDI (loves core work. "Feels so good when you can feel the muscles again!")

"Not in a crazy way, but I enjoy that it is *addicting."*

—SHELLEY (nearly stepped on a rattlesnake. "It scared the pee out of me.")

"Yes, for sure, when I was in my 20s. Now exercise is much more for balance and sanity."

—TRACY (most effective cross-training: sun salutations in yoga.)

"I was anorexic in high school, so I use exercise to eat what I want and not feel guilty. I have to work out a certain amount a week or I get stressed."

—BRIGITTE (favorite run: a new one.)

"I have definitely felt addicted to running, but not in an unhealthy way. It's just part of my life, and if I go without it for too long, I get grumpy."

—JILL (worst part of running: having to go Number Two on a run.)

> *"In college, when I first started running, I was quite addicted because it helped me drop the weight I had packed on my freshman year. I was running 6 miles a day, 6 days a week. On that seventh day, you didn't want to be around me. I felt extremely guilty and fat on those days, like I was letting my entire fitness regimen and health fall apart in those 24 hours."*
>
> —TAMARA (solves the world's problems on runs with her husband.)

so on) in the TV room. And, of course, I had to go hard or long after a day or two of easy or shorter workouts. Looking back over my fairly detailed notes, an average week included a little over 8 hours of exercise.

My borderline addiction began with an unexpected divorce. I had to fill previously occupied hours, or I'd wander around my empty house, crying my eyes puffy. Once I got rolling, the main reason I didn't skip a day of running, swimming, biking, or strength training was that I was afraid that if I took one day off, it would lead to two. Then two days would become a week of sloth, which would become two weeks, then a month, until I turned into a full-fledged slug. Becoming completely inactive would be problematic for several reasons, including boredom and loss of identity. Exercising was my main hobby. I guess I could have read even more voraciously, needlepointed more pillows, or cultivated other hobbies, but I didn't have any desire to take up watercoloring or become a philatelist.

I had spent my childhood days reading the *Little House on the Prairie* series and building gnome-homes out of bark and moss, so my fear was—actually is (who's kidding who? I should be speaking in the present tense)—that I'd revert to that natural state. I had evolved into an active, outdoorsy woman, and I wanted to remain one. And even though I've never battled my weight, I also am concerned that if exercise were taken out of the equation, the numbers on the scale would scurry up. My appetite is hearty. Or, as my rowing teammate Meg said to me in college, "Sarah, it's great how much food you eat, even in front of guys."

During The Streak, I also became addicted to the mental side of exercise. As in, "I go *mental* when I don't get in a good sweat." It starts with a slightly restless feeling in my limbs, which fuels a playback loop in my head of, "No workout yet today. No workout yet today." I've never tried heroin or meth, but when I watch movies with a druggie like Anne Hathaway's character in *Rachel Getting Married*, I can relate. Agitation fuels a jittery feeling in my belly, and my needle-to-the-vein cure is slipping on a sports bra and a pair of sneaks and hitting the pavement or the gym.

I come by this affliction naturally. Until recently, my now-83-year-old dad swam every single day. I remember when, on a business trip, he visited me in San Francisco. Before his arrival, when I told him I had found a public pool with convenient lap times, he chuckled and assured me, "Oh, I don't need to swim while I'm out there." Famous last words. On his first day, after brunch and a visit to the art museum, around 4 P.M., my dad looked like a caged animal. Pent-up energy had him reverberating like a tuning fork. I barely coughed out the line, "Do you want me to drive you to the pool?" before he exclaimed, "Yes!"

I laugh about my dad's obsessive behavior, yet my own actions weren't funny to me. The most twisted thing I ever did to ensure I got in a sweat session? Take your pick. Option A: Waking up at 3:30 A.M. to go for a 45-minute run before flying cross-country. I never knew a city could be so dark and desolate. As I ran along San Francisco's Marina Green, the only sound of life was the moan of a fog horn. Option B: Going for a power walk after work in February in Wellesley, a Boston suburb. Talk about dark! No streetlights, no sidewalks, the road was covered with rutted snow that had iced over, and it was about 15 degrees. Yet there I was, trying to walk 14-minute miles, pumping my arms like a locomotive. I vote for Option B. After all, I was able to sleep on the flight from San Francisco to Boston in Option A.

Miraculously, I never got sick during this 6-year stint. (No kids to expose me to hordes of germs through countless slurpy kisses!) I didn't suffer any sidelining injuries, either, despite training for my first two marathons during The Streak. The fact I remained healthy despite my go-go-go mentality is one reason I don't believe I was truly addicted to exercise. I compare myself to a runner I know who completes four to six marathons each year and averages at least 60 miles per week. She is forever getting stress fractures, muscle strains, and overuse injuries. Yet she runs right through them or, more aptly, *hobbles* through them, unwilling to change her clearly destructive behavior.

She subsists on a few PowerBars and an apple a day, which also points to issues way beyond checking off a moderate daily workout. As I mentioned, I'm a semi-pro eater. I often have two-course breakfasts, starting with steel-cut oatmeal mixed with yogurt and sliced almonds and finishing with toast or half of a bagel. I realize exercise addiction is not the same thing as an eating disorder, but among women I know, the two seem to go hand in hand. It's hard to say which is the horse and which is the cart, but during my 6-year stint, I often told myself I didn't have a problem because I had fat to spare.

It took a 3-month, world-tour honeymoon with Jack, my second husband, to break me of my exercise habit. Somewhere between Madrid and Mongolia, I realized that if I insisted on keeping The Streak going and skipped cathedral tours in favor of a sweat session, I'd return home without him. Jack doesn't share my commitment to exercise, so maintaining my log would have caused more friction than a hot 18-miler. The Louvre or laps? I chose love and culture over exercise.

But like Obama occasionally sneaking a cig outside the White House, I backslide every so often. Self-imposed rest is a concept I have a hard time embracing. Even though I'm well versed in the rationale for taking a day off—giving broken-down muscles the time to repair and grow stronger and preventing mental burnout or boredom—my subconscious craving for a workout nearly always wins the battle. I know it would be better for my body, and I might even become more fit if I gave it a chance to recover, but I just can't scale back. I often go weeks without a break and then take one only because life interrupts, like a long travel day (no more 3:30, pre-flight alarms for me) or a day full of family obligations.

Ironically, I am better at taming my exercise junkie tendencies when I'm training for a half-marathon or a full one. Something about being on a prescribed, written-out schedule makes it mentally easier for me to justify a rest day. Knowing in advance I will not exercise on Mondays helps keep the itchy-twitchy feeling at bay at the start of my workout week. Since it's the day after a long Sunday run, I feel almost as if I banked two workouts in one day. But one day off is more than enough: I'm raring to go for my track workouts on Tuesday mornings.

When I wrote about the topic of exercise addiction on my blog, debating whether I needed a twelve-step program for it, two readers shared an interesting theory, which I like: that humans, and especially women, used to be much more active than we are now. Today, we have machines to clean our clothes, dishes, and homes, and therefore we have leftover energy. "We were made to move, every day. Our bodies work better that way," one reader wrote. "You're used to it now, so you feel unsettled physically and psychologically if you skip it."

Scientific justifications aside, holding a proverbial mirror up to myself while writing this chapter has let me see I am obsessed with working out, which I qualify as a milder form of exercise addiction. I don't have to go for hours, and I don't have to go intensely, but I do have to go.

I dug up my old yellow sheets of paper, smoothed out the folds, and read over them. "3/26/06 Sunny bike ride through Weston. (Didn't push it too hard.) 75 minutes. 3/27/06 Swam at Regis. 20 fast 50s, alternating kick–pull–free. Felt good in H_2O. 2,200 yards. 55 minutes. 3/28/06 Ran on treadmill, then upper-body weights. 65 minutes." I was alternately fascinated and appalled. My behavior didn't seem so out of whack back then. I was also horrified because I realize my habits haven't changed all that much. I don't have rules anymore, but, like I said, I seldom take a rest day. I hope in a few years I won't look back on this current time in my life—and the life of my young children—and shudder at how out of balance it was.

Perhaps it's a good thing I no longer keep written records of my workouts.

.2 STARS: THEY'RE NOT JUST LIKE US!
By Sarah

Don't get me wrong: I ogle photos of sweaty, bare-chested Matthew McConaughey or Jake Gyllenhaal as much as the next gal, but most shots of stars trotting along the Strand in Santa Monica make me want to gag, not drool. I know we marathon-moms are supposed to be a supportive tribe, but—call me crazy—I'm just not buying that Tori Spelling is a dedicated runner. And I don't want a picture of her trotting alongside her hubby to represent my beloved sport to 10 million or so readers.

And, so—drum roll—the top ten reasons why celebrities splashed across *USWeekly* and *Star* give running a bad name:

1 Low-rise sweats, cotton Juicy Couture tanks, and unzipped hoodies aren't standard-issue running gear.

2 Neither are yoga pants long enough to sweep the street behind you and a top better suited for a self-conscious 11-year-old with breast buds, which is what Katie Holmes wore in the New York City Marathon.

3 And sunglasses with lenses as big as salad plates are definitely not the sign of a serious runner.

4 Wait, let's not forget the footwear: Pumas designed for kicking back, not running. Shoes that offer about as much support and cushioning as a flip-flop.

5 Really? You need a trainer to run next to you and carry your water for 3 whole miles?

6 What should jiggle a bit on their bodies—boobs and (facial) cheeks—usually appear rock-solid, thanks to a little extra silicone.

7 While their trucker hats and aforementioned ridiculous glasses send a don't-notice-me message, they look directly into the lenses of the paparazzi's cameras.

8 They never look like they're running at a challenging pace or even breathing hard.

9 When they do race, it's always a big-name event, where they're likely to be noticed, like the Malibu Triathlon or the New York City or London marathons. They aren't toeing the line at the local turkey trot.

10 And then there they are, in the next issue, lounging poolside or dining al fresco, cigarette in hand.

25

POTTY TALK: **PEEING, POOPING, PASSING GAS, AND PERIODS**

By Sarah

My first ultrasound. I couldn't wait. The high-tech look inside my belly, then 14 weeks into the 40-week journey, would make my pregnancy seem real. Until then, I wasn't convinced I actually had a fetus growing. It could've as easily been gas and bloating making my pants insanely uncomfortable by the end of the workday. Obeying doctor's orders, I gulped down copious amounts of water before heading over to the hospital for the procedure. Sitting in the waiting room, I had images of Huck Finn and Jim floating through my head: I was a raft, and my bladder was the dammed-up Mississippi.

At last my name was called, and Jack and I followed the ultrasound technician back to the examination room. I shuffled along, the pressure on my bladder nearly causing paralysis. I was in agony, yet I felt ridiculously proud I'd showed up with a "very full bladder," per instructions. Oh, Ms. Overachiever: The tech said my bladder was too full, obstructing her view of our little peanut. As I crept off the table to the restroom to release the floodgates, she said she'd never seen a woman with such an enormous bladder. As much as I love praise, this wasn't the type of compliment I was aiming for.

When I came out of the bathroom 3 minutes later, there was a gaggle of nurses standing around to get a look at me. Turns out the tech couldn't resist telling them about me. I felt I should be in the freak show. "Step right up, folks: Here's Calliope, a real live mermaid; Ferdinand, a 400-pound man who can swallow swords; and Sarah, the Woman with the Gigantic Bladder!"

Why am I oversharing like this? As proof I have a large storage capacity for urine. Yet still, I've had to relieve myself mid-run many a time. The fact that I live in a major metropolitan area doesn't prevent me from copping a squat along the way. My most recent release was between a dumpster and some bushes over near the twins' preschool. During daylight hours. Not exactly proud of it, but I don't really have a problem with it, either.

I'm not alone. Diana, a former co-worker, admitted to ducking behind parked cars about every mile in San Francisco's houses-stacked-on-top-of-each-other Noe Valley while running during her three pregnancies. Christine, a mom of two, is another fan of running for cover behind vehicles. "It's a last, but quick, resort," she told me. Her car-cover of choice? Little cars like a Mini Cooper, "because you can hide behind one and watch out its windows for passers-by at the same time."

Runners in more bucolic areas also answer the call of nature during a run: Jo, another mom of two, was running in upstate New York while visiting relatives, and she had to go. She thought she was in the woods, but it turned out to be someone's side yard. Not a recommended way of scoring points with in-laws.

Obviously I'm not shocked by any of these anecdotes, but I get the sense some women runners would be. Dimity and I have heard from a bunch of marathon moms who say they've never had to answer the call of nature while out on the road. Never? Is your bladder a bigger freak than mine? "I rarely have to pee," testified Holly, a mom of two, echoing countless similar comments. Now this I find remarkable, probably because I am borderline-obsessed with staying well hydrated.

I can't stand to be thirsty—or even anticipate being thirsty. The hardest thing I had to endure with the C-section delivery of our twins was the overwhelming thirst I experienced afterward. I tried to slip a nurse a $20 to smuggle me in a drink. My Oliver Twist–worthy pleas eventually wore down one sympathetic nurse, and she brought me a glass of watered-down grape juice with crushed ice. It was as heavenly as sipping a Mai Tai on a Tahitian beach with swimsuit-clad Daniel Craig.

But, wait, where was I?

Right, peeing by the side of the road. If you stay properly hydrated and go on runs longer than 2 hours, eventually you're going to have to make a pit stop. Certainly ducking into a gas station or McDonald's is an option, but in residential areas, it can be tough to find a bathroom that doesn't have bark for its décor or grass on its floor. So you have to suck it up; don't let a little thing like modesty get in the way. I have a philosophy about dropping trou in public: Folks are more embarrassed to see my butt than I am to have them see it. I'm not saying I think my ass rivals Jessica Biel's booty, but just that I feel most people are so shocked when they spy a bare bottom, they don't critique it for firmness or shape.

Which brings me to one of the many reasons why I love running skirts with spankies (modest, attached briefs) rather than a compression shorts-style liner underneath. Unlike their longer cousins, which need to be pulled down for clearance, spankies can be quickly pulled aside, allowing modesty during elimination. Case in point: I recently peed in downtown Portland in some bushes behind a U-Haul at the annual Doggie Dash. (Hey, if hundreds of dogs were relieving themselves in the vicinity, why couldn't I?) My Hood to Coast teammate Alexa would approve: Due in part to poor bladder control caused by the birth of her twin sons, she admits to being known as "Piss Pants" by her fellow runners. She told me, "I have been able to perfect my squatting technique so that I can pee in 4 seconds flat. I hardly lose any time at all!"

Jokes aside, Alexa's situation brings up a serious matter familiar to many runners, especially pregnant ones and moms who have destroyed their pelvic floor muscles: urinary incontinence. The leaking some moms experience on their first few runs post-partum doesn't always go away, like with Jill, a mother of three. Two years after the birth of second child, she was still leaking urine on her runs. Her innovative solution: "I just wear a pad when I run and keep going!"

A pee-pad sounds to me like a stopgap measure, not a long-term solution. If you have incontinence while running (or, heck, when you laugh, sneeze, or jump rope in kickboxing class), tell your OB/GYN. If the situation is beyond the scope of regular Kegels, she may refer you to a physical therapist, as mine did after the vaginal delivery of my older daughter. I didn't have incontinence, but after I pushed for nearly 6 hours—yes, as long as the average school day—my doctor worried I might develop a control problem. To head off any problems down the road (or on the road), I paid a call to a female physical therapist.

Just in case you're lucky enough to be in this focus group, here's some info to prepare you for another of those oh-so-pleasant encounters under the draped sheet: Most physical therapists use biofeedback, positioning an internal probe (think: a plastic and metal tampon) or electrodes (on the perineum), which are attached to a computer, so you can see how hard you're working. You do variations of coochie-tightening exercises, like as many quick flutters as possible in 90 seconds or extended clenches, going for a PR in how long you can squeeze. Depending on the severity of the problem, expect to visit the physical therapist about four to eight times, with treatment spread out over several months. I snapped back after about 10 weeks, but I'm still trotting around with my oversized bladder.

OK, enough talk about Number One. Let's progress to the other scintillating three Ps: passing gas, pooping, and periods.

PASSING GAS

Of course, I never, ever pass gas when I exercise, but I hear a lot of runners do. All right, I admit, maybe once or twice I've let out a squeaker while I'm in my sneakers. It's one thing to let it rip when you're by yourself, but what about when you're racing or running with somebody else? Turns out both Dimity and I have been kidding ourselves with the same bogus rationale: that we're running away

TAKE IT *From* A MOTHER
HOW DO YOU ACE THE PORTA-POTTY LINE?

"Just find the line with mostly men. They are much faster than women."

—ALLYSON (runs to feel good, get great legs, and, as her husband says, "keep the cuckoo bird in the clock.")

"Take your own toilet paper and go to the porta-potty with no TP."

—IVANA (occasional post-run treat: almond milk latte and chocolate croissant.)

"Arrive late. Everyone has already used the porta-potties, and they are lined up ready to go. It's one advantage I've found to a late babysitter delaying me on race morning."

—MARY (goal for every race: to maximize what she has. "Conditions and my conditioning vary, so I run for effort, not time.")

"Don't assume honey buckets are the only option. If you're at a park, there may be a shorter line at the park bathroom or at a nearby open public building. Or think about it before you get to the race course: My posse stopped into a Hilton after we parked and were walking to a race."

—DIMITY (you know enough about me already.)

"Always go to the end ones. Believe it or not, no one wants them."

—MELISSA ("If I weren't running, I'd be thick.")

"Once you're running, avoid the porta-potties between miles 1 and 3: They're packed with runners who couldn't get through the pre-race lines. Also, avoid those near the water zones, as they're also pretty busy."

—JUNKO (hates peeing in the woods. "I always feel like a tick is going to latch itself to my bottom.")

from the smell and no one will notice it. So that means you'd never smell a fart on a race course, which, as my singed nose hairs can attest, is definitely not the case.

We also know we're not alone because while snooping around the Internet, we discovered bloggers have written entire posts about letting one rip while running. One blogger suggested faking an injury or needing to retie your shoes if you need to blow a beefie while in a group. That way, you can float a fart off to the side of the road, then catch up with your running buddies. One thing we know from personal experience: If you need to let one rip, don't try to hold it. That can sometimes lead to a noisier, bigger eruption of gas a few blocks later. Some women swear they can let a fart slowly sneak out, but that's up there with running a 5-minute mile: We just don't have that kind of talent.

After weighing the options, my new policy is to fire off one and then own up to it. Like I tell our kids to do when they, um, step on a duck: Just say, "Excuse me." We all know we fart, so let's just acknowledge it, ask for forgiveness, and keep on running away from it.

POOPING

As runners, we all know taking a dump ranks right up there with double-knotting your shoes on the list of things to do before a run. Many runners swear by drinking coffee or hot water before a run to get things moving. Others do jumping jacks or a short neighborhood lap: The up-and-down motion gets things moving, and they are still in the vicinity of their bathroom. Then they start their real run. Fortunately, I find my body just knows when I'm going to hit the road: On the mornings I run, I wake up and my colon is ready to rumble.

But sure, there have been runs where things get shaken loose, and I've had to pick up the pace to get home pronto. I laughed in solidarity over a tale from Cheryl, the mother of one daughter, who "once had to go Number Two in the bushes outside my dad's house because I couldn't get the door open in time," she says. "I was completely embarrassed but had no choice but to do it. I was just hoping no one would come up the drive while I was doing my business." Similarly, Kat, a mom of two in Colorado Springs, was running with her husband's boss's wife (got that?) and "desperately had to go Number Two. I just ran into a ditch," she remembers. "It was embarrassing, but she's been a runner for 35 years, so she's done it all."

I can relate to their dilemma: Just as my colon knows when I'm going running, it also knows when I'm within 100 feet of the toilet after I finish my run. I can be fine up until steps from the porcelain, then it's a mad dash to get the capris down in time.

The stress of a race plays havoc with our innards. You can think you've emptied the chute, yet 5 minutes later, you feel the urge to purge again. We don't have a solution for this, although mother-of-five Mary once had a coach tell her to "stay away from green" in the days leading up to the race. Seems the coach thought the roughage in lettuce, kale, spinach, and the like was too much for the system to handle. I'm not sure a registered dietitian would approve, but I figure it's worth sharing because it has usually worked for Mary, a veteran of "too many 5Ks and 10Ks to count," none of which, it seems, required an extended pit stop.

If you can't accept having to wait in the porta-potty line yet another time, follow the lead of Christine. This running coach and mother of two overshared with us—which we always love—so now we are passing her story along to you.

"OK. I know this may be gross. But since we are all moms here: I love my son's potty seat that he learned to 'go' on. It all happened innocently. I kept his portable little potty in the back of my car, in case he had an emergency. I arrived late to a race and had no clue where the restrooms were. With no time to spare, I decided to use the toddler toilet in the back. I set it on the floor of the back seat and did my thing. Luckily I have tinted windows. It was so easy, and it got me thinking. So, when I did a marathon about an hour's drive from my house, I made sure to have the potty with me. I know this may be entirely too much info, but here goes: I took some plastic grocery bags to line the little potty so I could discard the you-know-what. Having that potty in my car saved me a ton of time, standing in the cold, waiting for a nasty porta-potty."

I'm fairly certain I couldn't squeeze my non-Biel buns between the railings of a toddler potty, so I'm stuck enduring the lines to—and stench of—the grown-up portable potties at races. But I totally applaud the innovative repurposing of one of the countless pieces of plastic necessary for childhood today.

PERIODS

How is a race like an outdoor wedding? In the weeks leading up to both of them, you pray the weather will be good—and you won't be having your period. At least that was me before the Eugene Marathon in 2009. It was rainy for the first few miles, but at least my uterine lining was firmly in place. I'll take it: One out of two ain't bad.

It does suck, though, to have your period during a race. You have to keep track of tampons that fill up faster than the kitchen sink, and potentially replace them mid-race, which means you need to somehow stash a new cooter plug on your person and find a bathroom for the switch out. A back-up pad gets all twisted and uncomfortable, especially those with "wings." (For whatever reason, they don't like to fly on running short liners.) Dehydration, and the accompanying headaches, seem to come on sooner than usual, and the cramps in your belly reverberate with the spasms in your legs, turning you into one massive running cramp. Not pretty.

Some women don't rely on prayers or luck. Instead, they use birth control to regulate their cycles. Several moms swear by the Mirena IUD, saying they haven't had their periods in the years since they started wearing one. Marathoner and mother-of-two Carmen "fiddles with birth control" so she is period-free during races. You didn't hear this from us—we're not medical professionals qualified to dole out such important advice—but skipping the "fake" pills in a birth control pack and instead jumping ahead to a new pack makes you skip a period that cycle.

Although messing with your hormones might be ill-advised, you may contemplate it after considering the plight of Jennifer, the mother of two boys. Poor gal: At about mile 5 of her very first race, Aunt Flo paid an unexpected visit. "And it was a half-marathon—I think I ran faster after that to hurry and finish the race! Yikes!" I'm hoping the added incentive netted her a long-standing PR. She at least deserves that.

Since we don't let a little thing like menstruation get in the way of our runs, some women have figured out the best line of protection. Here's helpful Coach Christine's advice: "I just use a super-size tampon and make sure to put a new one in as close as possible to the start of my run or race. Another thing I like to do is shorten the string, since it always seems to tug and bother me. So, after inserting, I tie a knot higher up and cut the string, usually to about half its length." (I was worried she might make a painful slip with the scissors, but Christine assured me, "It's not like my goods hang low.")

Tamara up in Seattle, mother of two, offered us some other super-valuable, albeit graphic, suggestions: "Make sure the tampon is good and stuck up there by running in place a bit before you leave home to make sure it's not sitting crooked or bent. Also, make sure the tampon string is not hanging out of your underwear or shorts liner, or caught in the skin fold located between your vagina and your leg. If it is, it could get pulled out, step-by-step, during your run."

Whatever route you choose to take, try your best to follow the lead of Brandi, a mother of a daughter. "My period drags me down a bit, but I know that running is what I need to perk me back up." And that boost is worth a little blood on any shorts liner.

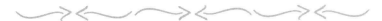

.2   PUBLIC SAFETY ANNOUNCEMENT
From Dimity

BEEP. BEEP. REALLY LOUD, ANNOYING BEEP.

We interrupt your regularly scheduled book to bring you the following announcement: Stay safe when you run.

Although I feel fairly invincible in my 6-foot, almost 4-inch frame, there have been times when I've doubted my safety while running. For example, the north end of Central Park, where the Central Park Jogger was raped and attacked in 1989 and a female runner was beaten to death in 1995, can give me the chills, especially when I realized I unknowingly ran near the latter's yet-undiscovered body. During a run on a semi-deserted road in Santa Fe, I ran over a bridge and saw a man below who was, um, servicing himself in broad daylight. (As I sped up, I threw up in my mouth.) On a run in Colorado Springs, I, hugging the curb, was nearly hit by a car—and then yelled at by the driver for assuming we could share the road.

If you accumulate enough miles under your shoes, stuff like that happens. Still, here are some ways to keep your runs as peaceful as possible:

♀ Keep your jewelry to a minimum.

♀ Carry or wear some kind of ID. If that's too high maintenance, write your name and home phone number on the tongue of your shoe.

♀ When you're running at dusk or dawn, make sure to have spots of reflectivity on your clothes and shoes. (No ugly traffic-cop vest necessary: Reflective armbands or tape that sticks to your clothes are as effective.)

♀ At intersections, make eye contact with drivers before you cross to make sure they see you. At times when I've run close to a car rolling through a stop sign, I've flung my arms out wide and yelled, "Do you see me?" It also helps to make eye contact with drivers of cars in motion who are headed toward you, sharing the lane. Doing so humanizes you, encouraging them to give you space.

♀ Run with a pal, especially in deserted or new areas.

♀ If you listen to music, keep the volume low enough so you can hear what's going on around you. Better yet: Keep it low and use only one earbud.

♀ Run tall and purposefully, make eye contact with fellow runners, and project a don't-mess-with-me 'tude. To an attacker, slumped shoulders, a shuffling step, and a downward gaze look exactly like an injured gazelle does to a lion: easy prey.

♀ Trust your intuition. If somebody shady approaches you asking for directions, don't stop. In this case, rudeness is called for.

♀ If you're (lucky enough to be) traveling alone, ask at the hotel front desk for a safe, well-populated route. (Write down the route and the address of the hotel, if you're prone to getting lost, like I am.) Then tell the valet or doorman when you expect to return.

This concludes the announcement. Please consult the Road Runners Club of America (rrca.org) for more tips and strategies. Thank you for your attention.

A FEW MORE REALLY LOUD, REALLY ANNOYING BEEPS.

26

THE **REAL** REASON WE RUN

Mile 26.

Even if you've never run a marathon, you've been there. You can hit it during your third week of running as a beginner, when the excited astonishment—*I can do this!*—that carried you through your first six runs has left the building. You can inch up to it on a hilly route, when all you see at the peak of a hard-won hill are many more to climb before you're home. You can dwell on it, after months off from running, thanks to a case of plantar fasciitis or a post-partum recovery period. And, of course, you can slam into it during a marathon.

Regardless of the situation in which you stare down your version of mile 26, one thing is a given: You have no clue how to conquer it. Every weapon you have—confidence, strength, momentum, sheer will—feels flimsy. Your quads, either real or proverbial, are tapped. Quite frankly, you are fed up with this running thing. What was wrong with chasing a little white ball around eighteen holes again?

Because you're a runner, you find a way to soldier through. You crank your tunes. You count your steps. You tell your buddy you are capital-H hurting and ask her to please just stay with you. You sign up for a 10K to jumpstart your training. You promise yourself if you get through this mile, you'll never make yourself run again (a promise we all know you'll never keep). Somehow, you keep moving forward.

The beauty of the mile 26s—no, that's not an oxymoron—lies not in their difficulty but in their simplicity. When all that's left is you and a challenge, running is distilled down to two things: putting one foot in front of the other and summoning a visceral feeling. Not the awful feelings of suffering and resistance as you gut it out, but the one that soars through you and almost carries you when you realize, *I've got this.*

The feeling swirls within you as you circle the track and traverse single-track trails. The feeling is the one that flushes your cheeks as you answer "yes" when somebody asks if you're a runner. The feeling taunts you when you're debating a run: *Do you crave me enough today to get out there?* The feeling gets mentioned frequently when you justify your running to your friends, husband, co-workers. The feeling hibernates in your soul when you take a break but is awakened as soon as you run a mile again. The feeling floods you when you cross a finish line.

The feeling is why you—and we—run, mile 26s and all. We guess we could live our lives without it, but we're not sure we'd want to.

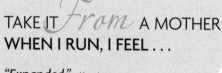

TAKE IT *From* A MOTHER
WHEN I RUN, I FEEL . . .

"Expanded."—Kami

"Happy."—Debbie

"Like my own person."—Molly

"Invigorated. Rejuvenated. Capable."—Angie

"Like I'm accomplishing something."—Kelly

"Calm."—Stephanie

"Free, empowered, and strong."—Christine

"Exhilarated."—Ellen

"Passionate and peaceful."—Jessica

"Energized."—Ashley

"Better than before I started."—Sheryl

"Elevated."—Dimity

"Relieved and refreshed."—Sari

"Good about myself."—Julie

"Amazing."—Mary

"Cleansed."—Christine

"Strong and sexy."—Susan

"Productive."—Cindy

"Relaxed."—Brigitte

"Satisfied."—Kelly

"Free."—Emily

"Complete."—Alexa

"Euphoric."—Megan

"Powerful and beautiful."—Leslie

"Proud."—Sarah

ACKNOWLEDGMENTS

From **Dimity**:

I am so appreciative to Grant, who has never once said "no" when I ask him, "Can I go for a run tomorrow morning?" I love you dearly and thank you from the bottom of my heart. I'm equally grateful to Amelia and Ben, who always hug me no matter how sweaty I am and remind me, through hundreds of games of tag, that running is supposed to be fun.

A huge thanks to my 'rents, Muti, J-Berg, and Dad. You all cheer me on in your respective ways. And to my sisters, Megan and Sarah, who have accompanied me on all kinds of journeys. Up for a half-marathon to celebrate my 40th?

Thanks to Bay Anapol, who is my go-to girl for advice and much-needed compliments; to Ivana Bisaro and Abby Ruby, who have coaxed more speed out of my legs than I thought possible; Katherine Spicer, whom I hold up as the ideal running partner and friend; Courtney McGovern, who convinced me to join crew way back in the day; Kathy Morgenstern, who never failed to entertain me as we trained for our first marathon; and Dan Helmick, who humored me for plenty of slow miles before he became a seriously fast runner.

A huge hug to Sarah for being an amazing teammate and friend. We were warned that co-authoring a book is a rough, exhausting experience that can easily end a relationship. I'm so glad we proved them wrong.

From Sarah:

Even though I run away from them almost every morning for some revitalizing solitude, I trust my husband, Jack, and my kids, Phoebe, John, and Daphne, know how much I love and treasure them.

I am eternally grateful to my parents. They didn't give me any running genes, but they have heaped support on me as I've discovered my inner athlete.

Muchas gracias, Eva, the *abuela* to my children, who, despite the language barrier, gets my running and my races.

Lynn Jennings: Being able to see myself as a runner through your clear-sighted, infinitely experienced eyes had a profound effect on my psyche and my confidence. Our months training together for the Eugene Marathon are some of the most special of my life.

A big shout-out of thanks to all the gal-pals whom I have trotted alongside over the years: Beth Brewster, Julie Carter, Christy Collinson, Dorothy Cooney, Courtenay Labson, all my See Jane Run Hood to Coast teammates, and Ellison Weist.

Two friends stand out in my marathon memories: Stacy Whitman, who joined me for the last 10K of the majority of my marathons, and Kate Boyd, who was always there for me when my 26.2s took me through beautiful Golden Gate Park. Thank you both.

I am filled with gratitude and admiration for Dimity McDowell. Somewhere through the years, she morphed from my protégée to my mentor, but above all, she's a dear friend whom I love greatly.

And thanks to anyone who has ever yelled, "Go, Champy, Champy, go!"

From Dimity and Sarah:

We are so appreciative of our agent, Jane Dystel, for helping this book become a reality, and of Chris Schillig, our editor, for giving us latitude to be ourselves. And we heart Tish Hamilton, who got this whole party started and continues to be a good friend and great editor. Thanks to Winni Wintermeyer, whose picture of us captures the spirit of our book. We are also thankful to Lynn Jennings, Magdalena Lewy-Boulet, and Kristen Sullivan for your time and thoughtful comments on our manuscript.

Finally, we owe a massive debt of gratitude to the 100+ running mothers who took time from their crazy schedules to fill out our way-too-long survey. Your thoughtful, funny, honest responses let us know we were on the right track with this book. We only wish there was room for more of you. Thank you, thank you.